The New

ATKINS

MADE EASY

For SENIORS

Feel Young and Vibrant with the Atkins Diet || Over 61 Delicious, Nutritious & Simple Recipes for Seniors

Dr. Jim Davis

CONTENTS

Chapter 4: Delicious and Nutritious Atkins Diet Recipes for Seniors

LOW CARBS

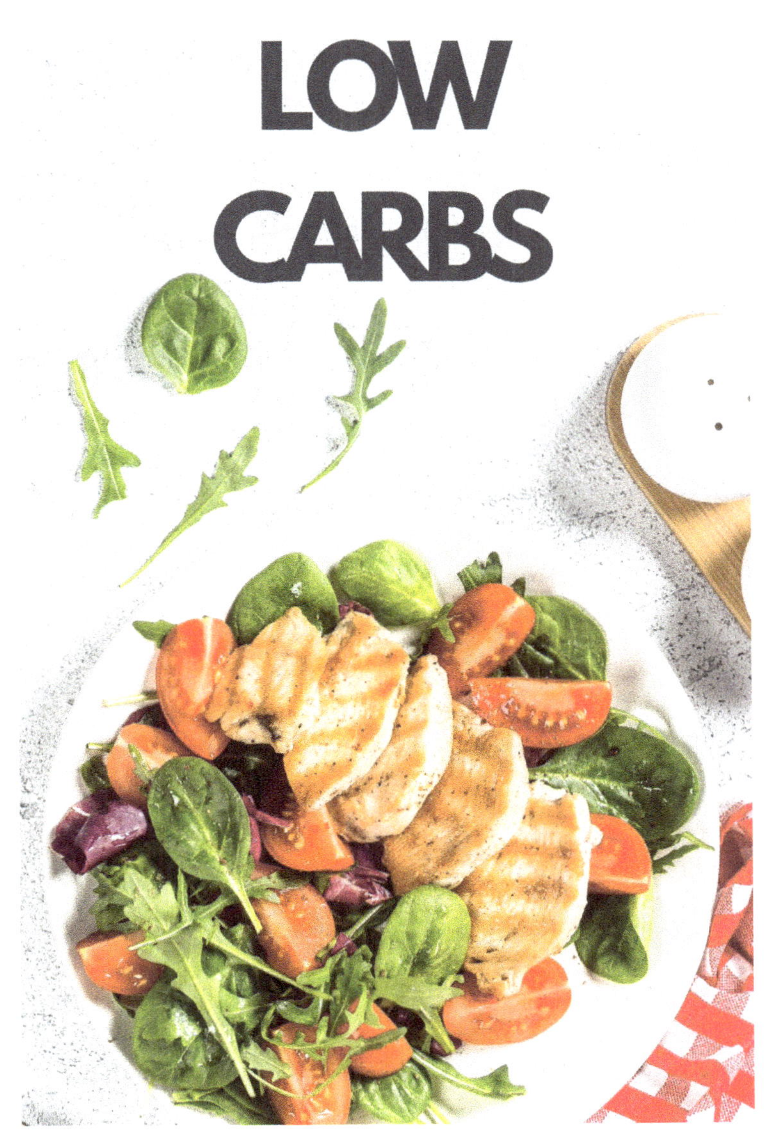

INTRODUCTION

Fifty-year-old Kristen had spent years feeling tired, sluggish, and dissatisfied with her health. Despite her best efforts, she struggled to find a diet that worked for her aging body – until she discovered "Atkins Diet Made Easy for Seniors" while browsing online.

Armed with the knowledge and recipes from the book, Kristen embarked on her Atkins journey with determination and hope. She found herself enjoying delicious meals that kept her feeling satisfied and energized throughout the day, all while shedding excess weight and improving her overall health.

Week by week, Kristen noticed remarkable changes in her body and mind. The aches and pains that had plagued her for years began to fade away, replaced by a newfound sense of vitality and well-being.

As she continued with the Atkins diet, she noticed that her joints felt better and she was able to do more of the activities that she enjoyed. She was even able to start walking and swimming again. She felt great and was so happy that she had found a way to be healthy while still enjoying the foods that she loved. She knew that the Atkins diet was more than just a diet; it was a lifestyle that had given her a new lease on life.

As we age, it's crucial to prioritize our health and well-being, and what better way to do so than with a diet that promotes weight loss, improved energy levels, and better overall health?

In this book, you'll find everything you need to know to get started on your Atkins journey, tailored specifically for seniors. Whether you're looking to shed those stubborn pounds, boost your energy levels, or simply improve your overall health, the Atkins diet offers a flexible and sustainable approach to achieving your goals.

With this book as your guide, you'll be empowered to take control of your health and transform your life for the better. Say goodbye to fad diets and restrictive eating plans – it's time to embrace a healthier, happier you with the Atkins diet.

CHAPTER ONE

The Principle of the Atkins Diet

The popular low-carb diet known as the Atkins Diet was created in the 1960s by Robert C. Atkins, a cardiologist. The Atkins Diet emphasizes protein and fats while limiting carbohydrates. There are various stages to the Atkins Diet for maintaining and losing weight. An extremely low-carb diet is the first step. The Atkins Nutritional Approach is the official name of the Atkins Diet. It is widely discussed in books and is recognized as the origin of the low-carb movement.

The Atkins Diet aims to alter your eating patterns so that you can lose weight and keep it off. The Atkins Diet claims to be a healthy way of eating for the rest of your life. It claims that it's a healthy strategy for improving health issues like metabolic syndrome or high blood pressure, losing weight, or increasing energy.

Eating the proper proportion of fats, proteins, and carbs is the fundamental nutritional goal of the Atkins Diet in order to achieve the best possible weight loss and health.

The Atkins Diet blames the conventional low-fat, high-carb American diet for obesity and related health issues like type 2 diabetes and heart disease. According to the Atkins Diet, you don't have to stay away from fatty meat cuts or remove extra fat. What matters is to regulate carbohydrates instead.

Eat too many carbohydrates, especially sugar, white flour, and other refined carbohydrates, according to the Atkins Diet, and you'll have a lot of problems. According to the Atkins Diet, it causes weight gain, blood sugar abnormalities, and heart issues. Therefore, the Atkins Diet restricts carbohydrates. A diet high in fat and protein is recommended by the Atkins Diet. Yet according to the Atkins Diet, it's not a high-protein diet.

The Atkins Diet is constantly evolving, much like many diet regimens. It now promotes consuming more veggies high in fiber and has been updated to accommodate vegan and vegetarian diets. It also covers health issues that may surface when a low-carb diet is first adopted.

The Phases of the Atkins Diet

There are four stages to the Atkins Diet. You can begin at any point during the first three phases, depending on your weight-loss objectives.

Phase 1: Induction

You eliminate nearly all carbohydrates from your diet during this strict phase. Merely 20 grams of net carbohydrates are consumed daily, primarily from vegetables. Rather than obtaining approximately 50% of your daily energy from carbohydrates, as suggested by the majority of nutrition guidelines, you only obtain roughly 10%. "Foundation" veggies like peppers, green beans, celery, cucumber, asparagus, and broccoli should make up 12 to 15 grams of your daily net carb intake.

You consume protein-rich foods at every meal during this phase, such as meat, eggs, cheese, poultry, and fish and shellfish. Limiting oils and fats is not necessary. However, most fruits, baked items with added sugar, breads, pastas, cereals, nuts, and alcohol are off limits. You have eight glasses of water or more each day. Depending on your rate of weight reduction, you spend at least two weeks in this phase.

Phase 2: Balancing

You continue to consume at least 12 to 15 grams of net carbohydrates per day from foundation veggies during this phase. You continue to abstain from meals that have added sugar. As you continue to lose weight, you can gradually reintroduce some nutrient-dense carbohydrates, like additional veggies, berries, nuts, and seeds. This phase lasts until you're approximately 10 pounds (4.5 kg) away from your target weight.

Phase 3: Pre-maintenance

During this stage, you gradually broaden your diet to include more fruits, whole grains, and veggies. You can increase your weekly intake of carbohydrates by roughly 10 grams. But if you don't lose weight, you have to cut back. This phase lasts until the desired weight is attained.

Phase 4: Lifetime maintenance

Once you hit your target weight, you enter this phase. After that, you continue eating in this manner forever.

The Health Benefits of the Atkins Diet

The Atkins Diet has a number of potential health benefits that includes;

1.   *Weight loss:* By limiting carbohydrate intake, the Atkins Diet can promote weight loss by encouraging the body to burn fat for fuel instead of carbohydrates. This can lead to significant initial weight loss, especially in the first few weeks of the diet.

2.   ***Improved blood sugar control:*** By reducing carbohydrate intake, the Atkins Diet can help stabilize blood sugar levels, which is beneficial for individuals with diabetes or insulin resistance. This can lead to better overall blood sugar control and reduced risk of complications.

3.   ***Reduced risk of heart disease:*** While the Atkins Diet was initially controversial due to its high fat content, research has shown

that it can actually improve several risk factors for heart disease, including blood pressure, triglyceride levels, and HDL cholesterol levels.

4. *Increased satiety:* Foods high in protein and healthy fats tend to be more filling than those high in carbohydrates, which can help reduce appetite and prevent overeating. This can make it easier to adhere to the Atkins Diet and maintain weight loss over the long term.

5. *Improved lipid profile:* Despite being high in saturated fat, the Atkins Diet has been shown to improve the lipid profile in some individuals by increasing HDL cholesterol

(the *"good"* cholesterol) and decreasing triglycerides.

6. ***Better energy levels:*** Many people report feeling more energetic and alert on the Atkins Diet, likely due to more stable blood sugar levels and reduced reliance on carbohydrates for energy.

CHAPTER TWO

The Benefits of the Atkins Diet for Seniors

As individuals age, maintaining optimal health becomes increasingly important for a vibrant and fulfilling life. Among the various dietary approaches available, the Atkins Diet stands out as a compelling option for seniors. While this diet has been popularized for its weight loss benefits, its advantages extend beyond just shedding pounds, particularly for seniors. With this, we will explore the benefits of the Atkins Diet specifically tailored to the needs and concerns of older adults.

1. Weight Management

Seniors often struggle with maintaining a healthy weight due to factors such as decreased metabolism and decreased physical activity. The Atkins Diet can be beneficial for seniors in managing their weight effectively. By reducing carbohydrate intake and emphasizing protein and healthy fats, the Atkins Diet helps seniors feel full and satisfied while consuming fewer calories, making it easier to achieve and maintain a healthy weight.

2. Improved Blood Sugar Control

Seniors are at a higher risk of developing type 2 diabetes or experiencing fluctuations in blood sugar levels. The Atkins Diet focuses on limiting carbohydrates, which can help stabilize blood sugar levels and reduce the risk of insulin resistance. For seniors with diabetes or prediabetes, following the Atkins Diet under the guidance of a healthcare professional can lead to better blood sugar control and potentially reduce the need for medication.

3. Enhanced Cognitive Function

Cognitive decline is a common concern among seniors, with conditions such as Alzheimer's disease and dementia becoming more prevalent as individuals age. Research suggests that diets high in refined carbohydrates may contribute to cognitive impairment and decline. In contrast, the Atkins Diet emphasizes foods rich in omega-3 fatty acids, antioxidants, and other nutrients that support brain health. By reducing carbohydrate intake and incorporating brain-boosting foods, the Atkins Diet may help seniors maintain cognitive function and reduce the risk of cognitive decline.

4. Cardiovascular Health

Heart disease remains a leading cause of mortality among seniors, making cardiovascular health a top priority for this demographic. While early versions of the Atkins Diet were criticized for their high saturated fat content, newer iterations emphasize the importance of healthy fats, such as those found in avocados, nuts, and olive oil. By prioritizing these heart-healthy fats and lean protein sources, the Atkins Diet can help seniors improve their lipid profiles, lower blood pressure, and reduce the risk of cardiovascular disease.

5. Increased Energy Levels

Fatigue and low energy levels are common complaints among seniors, often attributed to age-related changes in metabolism and hormone levels. The Atkins Diet provides a steady source of energy by stabilizing blood sugar levels and promoting the use of fat stores for fuel. As seniors adapt to the Atkins Diet, many report experiencing increased energy levels, allowing them to engage in daily activities with greater ease and enjoyment.

6. Preservation of Muscle Mass

Sarcopenia, or age-related muscle loss, is a significant concern for seniors, as it can lead to decreased strength, mobility, and independence. Adequate protein intake is essential for preserving muscle mass, and the Atkins Diet emphasizes protein-rich foods such as meat, fish, eggs, and dairy products. By prioritizing protein consumption and incorporating resistance training exercises, seniors can maintain or even build muscle mass while following the Atkins Diet, supporting overall physical function and vitality.

7. Joint Health

Arthritis and other joint-related conditions are prevalent among seniors and can significantly impact mobility and quality of life. The Atkins Diet may offer benefits for joint health due to its anti-inflammatory properties. By reducing consumption of refined carbohydrates and processed foods, which can contribute to inflammation in the body, seniors following the Atkins Diet may experience reduced joint pain and stiffness, allowing for greater comfort and mobility.

CHAPTER THREE

Getting Started on the Atkins Diet

Getting started on the Atkins Diet is like embarking on a journey to discover a new way of eating—one that prioritizes wholesome, nutrient-dense foods while reshaping your body's metabolism. Imagine stepping into a world where you bid farewell to the constant cravings for sugary treats and starchy snacks, and instead, embrace a satisfying array of proteins, healthy fats, and vibrant vegetables. It's about redefining your relationship with food and fueling your body in a way that promotes sustained energy and vitality.

At the heart of the Atkins Diet lies a simple yet powerful concept: by reducing your intake of carbohydrates and increasing consumption of protein and healthy fats, you can effectively shift your body into a state of ketosis, where it burns fat for fuel. It's a metabolic transformation that holds the key to unlocking your body's natural fat-burning potential, leading to weight loss and improved overall health.

It's about letting go of the notion that fat is the enemy and embracing it as a valuable source of energy and satiety. It's also about recognizing the importance of balance and variety in your meals, ensuring that you nourish your body with a diverse range of nutrients to support optimal health.

Dealing with common challenges during the induction phase

For seniors embarking on the induction phase of the Atkins Diet, there are several common challenges to navigate, but with tailored strategies, these obstacles can be effectively managed to ensure a successful transition to a low-carbohydrate lifestyle.

One significant challenge you may face is adjusting to the drastic reduction in carbohydrate intake. Many seniors have been accustomed to diets rich in carbohydrates throughout their lives, making it difficult to suddenly restrict these foods. To address this, you can gradually reduce your carbohydrate intake before officially starting the induction phase. This gradual approach can help ease the transition and minimize feelings of deprivation.

Another challenge you may encounter is the potential for side effects such as fatigue, headaches, and constipation as your body adapt to ketosis. But then, you should prioritize hydration by drinking plenty of water throughout the day, as dehydration can exacerbate these symptoms. Additionally, seniors can increase their intake of electrolyte-rich foods like avocados, nuts, and leafy greens to help replenish electrolyte levels and alleviate discomfort.

It may be challenging to navigate social situations and dining out while adhering to the strict guidelines of the induction phase. To overcome this, you can plan ahead by researching restaurant menus or suggesting low-carb meal options to friends and family when dining together. Bringing a homemade dish to social gatherings ensures there's always a suitable option available.

You may encounter concerns about the safety and effectiveness of the Atkins Diet, especially if you have pre-existing health conditions or taking medications. It's crucial for you to consult with your healthcare provider before starting any new diet or making significant dietary changes. A healthcare professional can provide personalized guidance and ensure that the Atkins Diet is appropriate for your health needs.

Successful strategies for sticking to the Atkins Diet

Sticking to the Atkins diet as a senior can be achieved through several successful strategies tailored to your lifestyle and needs.

- *Focus on planning your meals ahead of time:* This involves creating a weekly meal plan that includes a variety of low-carb foods such as lean proteins, vegetables, and healthy fats. By having a structured meal plan, you can ensure you have the necessary ingredients on hand and avoid temptation.

• *Prioritize portion control and mindful eating:* As a senior, your metabolism may have slowed down, so it's important to be mindful of portion sizes to avoid overeating. Pay attention to hunger and fullness cues to prevent unnecessary snacking or indulging in high-carb foods.

• *Find alternatives for your favorite high-carb foods:* Experiment with low-carb substitutes for pasta, bread, and sweets to satisfy cravings without derailing your progress on the Atkins diet.

• *Incorporate fiber-rich foods:* Include plenty of fiber-rich foods like leafy greens and nuts in your diet. These not only contribute to a sense of fullness but also support digestion, addressing specific concerns that may arise for seniors.

- ***Stay hydrated and stay active:*** Drinking plenty of water throughout the day can help curb cravings and keep you feeling energized. Regular physical activity, even gentle exercises like walking or yoga, can enhance weight loss and overall well-being while following the Atkins diet.

Tips for transitioning to the maintenance phase

Transitioning to the maintenance phase of the Atkins diet can be a gradual and rewarding process, especially for seniors looking to sustain their progress and enjoy long-term health benefits. Here are some tailored tips to help you navigate this phase successfully:

1. *Slow and Steady Approach:* Gradually increase your daily carbohydrate intake by adding small portions of healthy carbs, such as fruits, whole grains, and legumes. Monitor your body's response and adjust accordingly to maintain your desired weight and energy levels.

2. *Monitor Progress:* Keep track of your weight, energy levels, and overall well-being as you introduce more carbohydrates into your diet. Regular monitoring allows you to make informed adjustments and ensures you stay on track with your health goals.

3. *Focus on Whole Foods:* Emphasize whole, nutrient-dense foods in your diet, including lean proteins, vegetables, fruits, and healthy fats. These foods provide essential nutrients and support overall health while helping to maintain weight loss.

4. *Portion Control:* Continue practicing portion control to prevent overeating and maintain a healthy balance of macronutrients. Be mindful of serving sizes, especially when reintroducing higher-carb foods, to avoid unintentionally exceeding your carbohydrate intake.

5. *Stay Active:* Maintain a regular exercise routine to support weight management, muscle strength, and overall well-being.

Incorporate a variety of physical activities that you enjoy, such as walking, swimming, or gentle strength training, to stay active and mobile as a senior.

6. *Listen to Your Body:* Pay attention to how different foods make you feel and adjust your diet accordingly. Focus on eating intuitively and honoring your body's hunger and fullness cues to promote a healthy relationship with food.

7. *Seek Support:* Surround yourself with a supportive network of friends, family, or fellow Atkins dieters who can provide encouragement, accountability, and practical tips for navigating the maintenance phase successfully.

CHAPTER FOUR

Delicious and Nutritious Atkins Diet Recipes for Seniors

Spinach and Mushroom Omelette

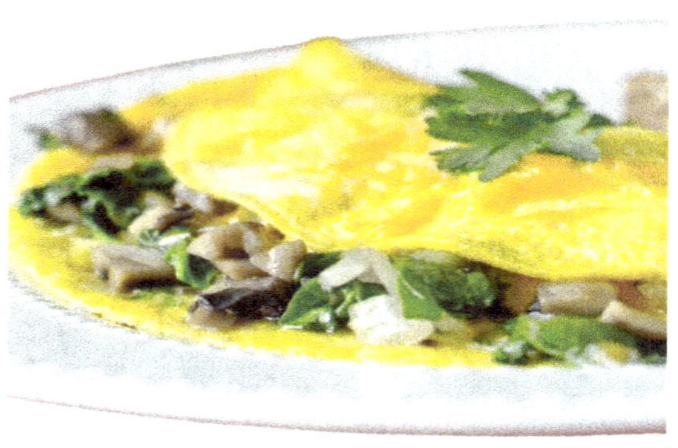

Cooking Time: 10 minutes

Servings: 2

Ingredients

- 4 large eggs
- 1 cup fresh spinach, chopped
- ½ cup mushrooms, sliced
- ¼ cup shredded cheddar cheese
- 2 tablespoons heavy cream
- Salt and pepper to taste
- 1 tablespoon olive oil

Procedure

1. In a bowl, whisk together the eggs, heavy cream, salt, and pepper until well combined.
2. Heat olive oil in a non-stick skillet over medium heat.

3. Add sliced mushrooms to the skillet and sauté until they release their moisture and become tender.

4. Add chopped spinach to the skillet and cook until wilted.

5. Pour the egg mixture over the vegetables in the skillet. Allow the edges to set, then gently lift with a spatula to let the uncooked egg flow underneath.

6. Sprinkle shredded cheddar cheese evenly over the omelette.

7. Once the omelette is mostly set but still slightly runny on top, fold it in half using the spatula.

8. Continue cooking until the cheese is melted, and the omelette is cooked to your desired level of doneness.

9. Slide the omelette onto a plate and serve hot.

Avocado and Bacon Breakfast Salad

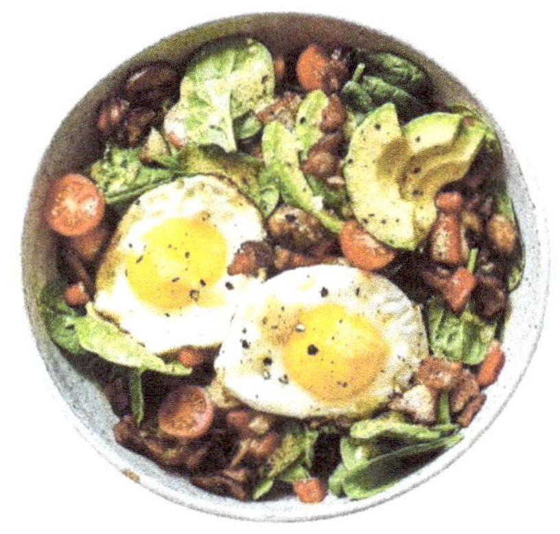

Cooking Time: 15 minutes

Servings: 2

Ingredients

- 4 slices bacon
- 2 large eggs

- 2 cups mixed salad greens
- 1 ripe avocado, diced
- ¼ cup cherry tomatoes, halved
- 2 tablespoons red onion, thinly sliced
- 2 tablespoons olive oil
- 1 tablespoon balsamic vinegar
- Salt and pepper to taste

Procedure

1. Cook the bacon in a skillet over medium heat until crispy. Remove from the skillet and drain on paper towels. Once cooled, crumble or chop the bacon into smaller pieces.
2. In the same skillet, fry the eggs to your desired level of doneness (e.g., sunny-side-up or over-easy).

3. In a large bowl, combine the mixed
   salad greens, diced avocado, halved
   cherry tomatoes, and thinly sliced red
   onion.
4. In a small bowl, whisk together the
   olive oil, balsamic vinegar, salt, and
   pepper to make the dressing.
5. Drizzle the dressing over the salad and
   toss gently to coat the ingredients
   evenly.
6. Divide the dressed salad among
   serving plates or bowls.
7. Top each serving with crispy bacon
   and a fried egg.
8. Season with additional salt and pepper
   if desired.

Smoked Salmon and Cream Cheese Roll-Ups

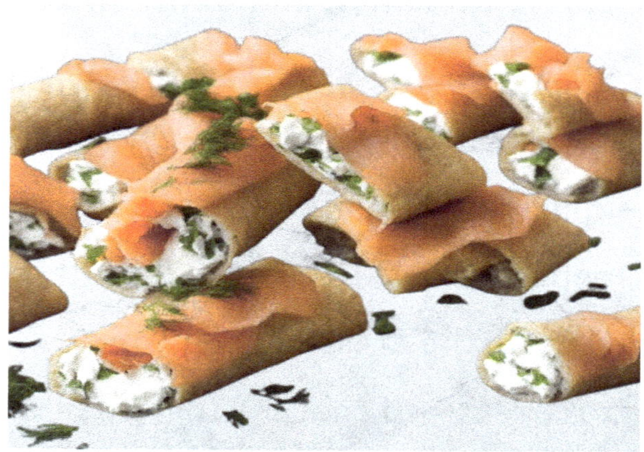

Preparation Time: 10 minutes

Servings: 2

Ingredients

- 4 ounces smoked salmon
- 4 ounces cream cheese, softened
- 1 tablespoon capers, drained
- 1 tablespoon fresh dill, chopped

- 1 tablespoon lemon juice
- Salt and pepper to taste
- Cucumber slices (optional, for serving)

Procedure

1. In a bowl, combine the softened cream cheese, chopped fresh dill, drained capers, and lemon juice. Mix well until all ingredients are incorporated.
2. Lay out the smoked salmon slices on a clean work surface.
3. Spread a thin layer of the cream cheese mixture evenly over each smoked salmon slice.
4. Season the cream cheese layer with salt and pepper to taste.

5. Carefully roll up each smoked salmon slice with the cream cheese mixture inside.

6. If desired, slice cucumber thinly lengthwise using a vegetable peeler or mandoline.

7. Serve the smoked salmon roll-ups as they are or wrap each roll-up in a cucumber slice for added freshness and crunch.

Vegetable Frittata

Cooking Time: 20 minutes
Servings: 4

Ingredients

- 6 large eggs
- ¼ cup heavy cream
- 1 cup mixed vegetables (such as bell peppers, onions, spinach, mushrooms), chopped
- ¼ cup shredded cheese (cheddar, mozzarella, or your choice)
- 2 tablespoons olive oil
- Salt and pepper to taste

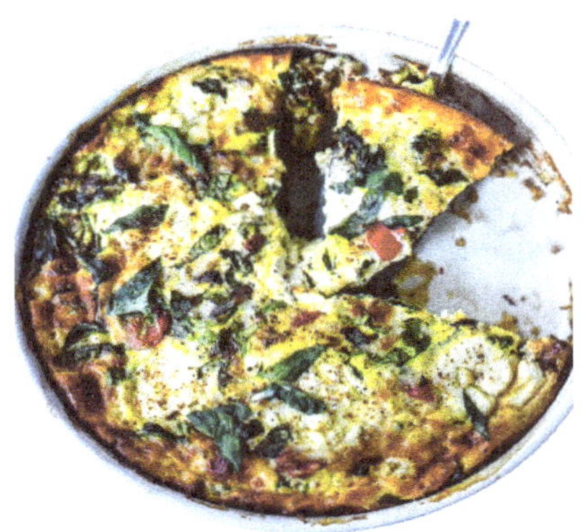

Procedure

1. Preheat your oven to 350°F (175°C).

2. In a bowl, whisk together the eggs and heavy cream until well combined. Season with salt and pepper to taste.

3. Heat olive oil in an oven-safe skillet over medium heat.

4. Add the chopped mixed vegetables to the skillet and sauté until they are tender, about 5-7 minutes.

5. Pour the egg mixture over the vegetables in the skillet. Gently stir to distribute the vegetables evenly.

6. Allow the frittata to cook on the stovetop for 3-4 minutes, or until the edges start to set.

7. Sprinkle the shredded cheese evenly over the top of the frittata.

8. Transfer the skillet to the preheated oven and bake for 10-12 minutes, or until the frittata is set and the cheese is melted and bubbly.
9. Remove the skillet from the oven and let the frittata cool for a few minutes.
10. Slice the frittata into wedges and serve warm.

Cottage Cheese and Berry Bowl

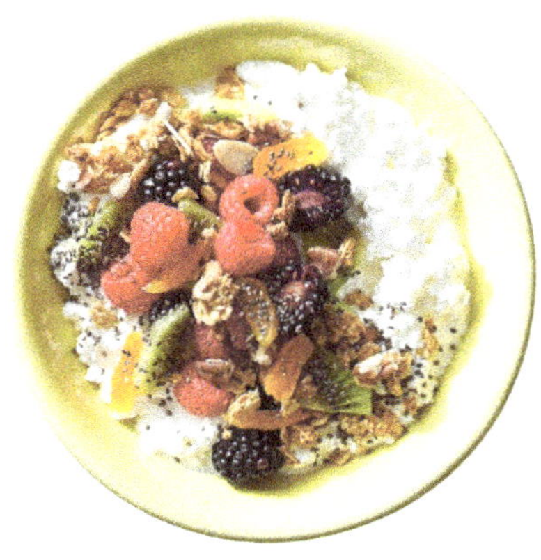

Preparation Time: 5 minutes

Servings: 1

<u>**Ingredients**</u>

- 1 cup cottage cheese (full-fat or low-fat)
- ½ cup mixed berries (such as strawberries, blueberries, raspberries)
- 1 tablespoon chopped nuts (such as almonds, walnuts, or pecans)
- 1 tablespoon unsweetened coconut flakes (optional)
- 1 teaspoon vanilla extract (optional)
- 1 teaspoon honey or low-carb sweetener (optional)

<u>**Procedure**</u>

1. In a bowl, combine the cottage cheese
   with the vanilla extract and honey or
   sweetener if using. Mix well to
   incorporate the flavors.
2. Wash the mixed berries and pat them
   dry with a paper towel.
3. If desired, slice larger berries such as
   strawberries into smaller pieces.
4. Spoon the sweetened cottage cheese
   into serving bowls.
5. Top the cottage cheese with the mixed
   berries, arranging them evenly over
   the surface.
6. Sprinkle chopped nuts and
   unsweetened coconut flakes over the
   berries for added texture and flavor.
7. Serve immediately and enjoy!

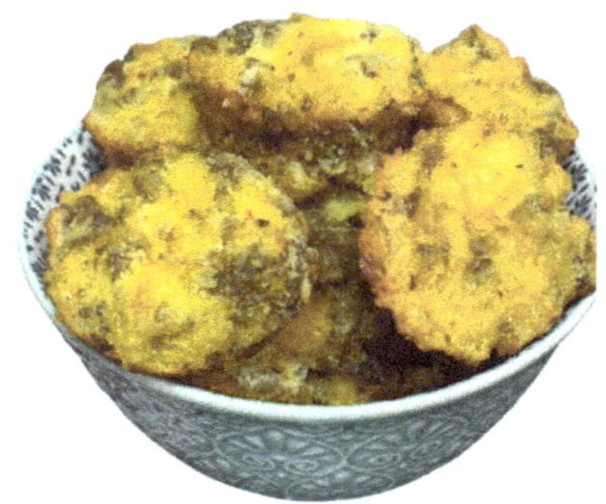

Cooking Time: 25 minutes

Servings: 12 muffins

Ingredients

- 8 ounces breakfast sausage, cooked and crumbled
- 1 cup almond flour
- 1 teaspoon baking powder
- ½ teaspoon garlic powder
- ½ teaspoon onion powder
- ¼ teaspoon salt
- ¼ teaspoon black pepper

- 4 large eggs
- ¼ cup unsalted butter, melted
- 1 cup shredded cheddar cheese

Procedure

1. Preheat your oven to 350°F (175°C). Line a muffin tin with paper liners or grease the cups with cooking spray.
2. In a large bowl, combine the almond flour, baking powder, garlic powder, onion powder, salt, and black pepper. Mix well to combine.
3. In another bowl, whisk the eggs and melted butter together until smooth.
4. Pour the egg mixture into the dry ingredients and stir until just combined.

5. Fold in the cooked and crumbled sausage and shredded cheddar cheese until evenly distributed throughout the batter.

6. Spoon the batter into the prepared muffin tin, filling each cup about 3/4 full.

7. Bake in the preheated oven for 20-25 minutes, or until the muffins are golden brown and a toothpick inserted into the center comes out clean.

8. Remove the muffins from the oven and allow them to cool in the pan for a few minutes before transferring to a wire rack to cool completely.

9. Serve the sausage and cheese muffins warm or at room temperature.

Coconut Chia Pudding

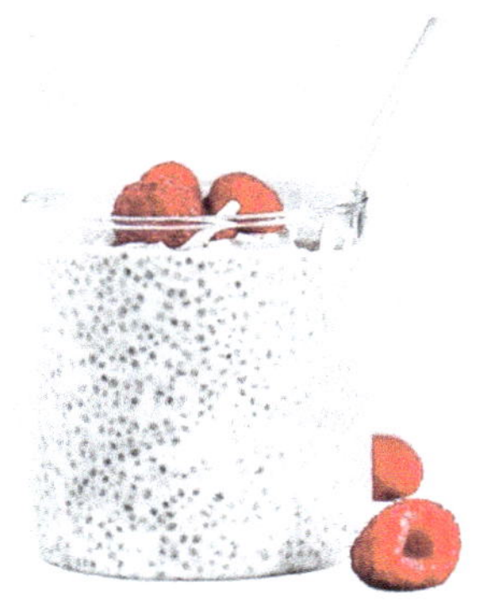

Preparation Time: 5 minutes (plus chilling time)

Servings: 2

Ingredients

- ¼ cup chia seeds
- 1 cup unsweetened coconut milk
- 1 tablespoon low-carb sweetener (such as stevia or erythritol)
- ½ teaspoon vanilla extract

Optional toppings: sliced strawberries, blueberries, almonds, unsweetened coconut flakes

Procedure

1. In a bowl or jar, combine the chia seeds, unsweetened coconut milk, low-carb sweetener, and vanilla extract.
2. Stir well to combine, making sure the chia seeds are evenly distributed throughout the mixture.
3. Cover the bowl or jar and refrigerate for at least 2 hours, or preferably overnight, to allow the chia seeds to absorb the liquid and thicken into a pudding-like consistency.
4. Once the chia pudding has set, give it a good stir to break up any clumps and distribute the pudding evenly.

5. Divide the chia pudding into serving bowls or glasses.

6. Top each serving with sliced strawberries, blueberries, almonds, and unsweetened coconut flakes, or any other toppings of your choice.

7. Serve the coconut chia pudding chilled and enjoy!

Salmon and Asparagus Bundles

Cooking Time: 15-20 minutes

Servings: 4

Ingredients

- 4 salmon fillets, about 4 oz each

- 1 bunch of asparagus, trimmed

- 2 tablespoons olive oil

- Salt and pepper to taste

- 1 lemon, thinly sliced

- 2 cloves garlic, minced

- Fresh herbs (such as parsley or dill) for garnish (optional)

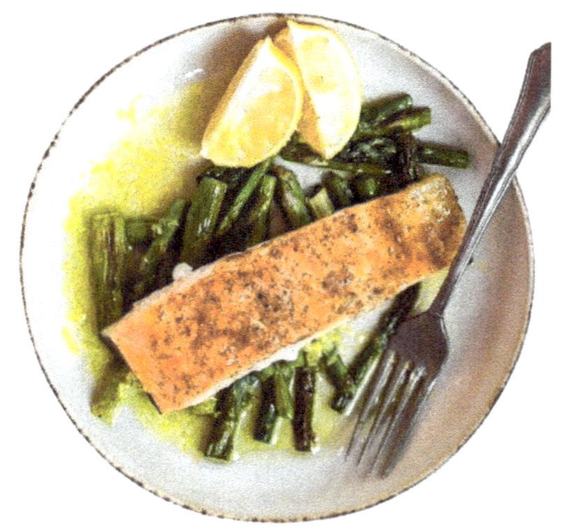

Procedure

1. Preheat your oven to 375°F (190°C).

2. Take a large piece of aluminum foil
   and fold it in half to create a sturdy
   base. Repeat to create four foil
   squares, large enough to wrap each
   salmon fillet and a handful of
   asparagus.

3. Place a salmon fillet in the center of
   each foil square. Season the salmon
   with salt, pepper, and minced garlic.

4. Arrange a handful of trimmed
   asparagus spears around each salmon
   fillet.

5. Drizzle olive oil over the salmon and
   asparagus bundles. Squeeze fresh
   lemon juice over each bundle and
   place a couple of lemon slices on top.

6. Carefully fold the sides of the foil up
   and over the salmon and asparagus,

sealing the edges tightly to create a packet.

7. Place the foil packets on a baking sheet and bake in the preheated oven for 15-20 minutes, or until the salmon is cooked through and the asparagus is tender.

8. Once cooked, carefully open the foil packets (watch out for steam) and transfer the salmon and asparagus to serving plates.

9. Garnish with fresh herbs, if desired, and serve hot.

Tuna Salad Stuffed Bell Peppers

Cooking Time: 20-25 minutes
Servings: 4

<u>**Ingredients**</u>

- 4 large bell peppers, any color

- 2 cans (5 oz each) of tuna, drained

- ½ cup mayonnaise

- ¼ cup diced celery

- ¼ cup diced red onion

- 1 tablespoon Dijon mustard

- Salt and pepper to taste

Optional toppings: shredded cheese, sliced olives, chopped parsley

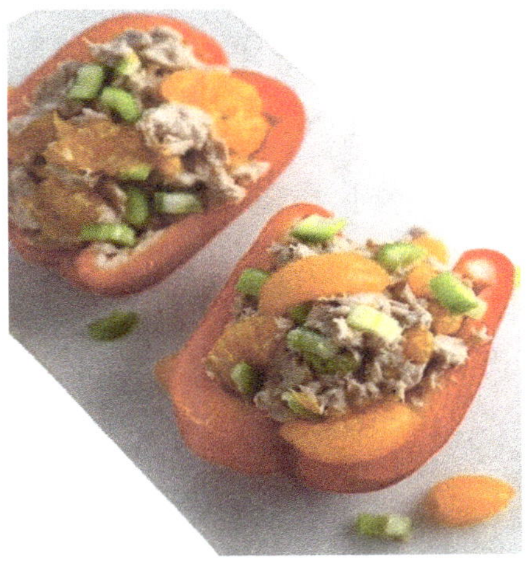

<u>**Procedure**</u>

1. Preheat your oven to 375°F (190°C).

2. Cut the tops off the bell peppers and remove the seeds and membranes from inside. Rinse the peppers under cold water and pat dry with paper towels.

3. In a mixing bowl, combine the drained tuna, mayonnaise, diced celery, diced red onion, and Dijon mustard. Season with salt and pepper to taste. Mix until well combined.

4. Stuff each bell pepper with the tuna salad mixture, pressing down gently to pack it in.

5. Place the stuffed bell peppers in a baking dish, standing upright.

6. Optional: sprinkle shredded cheese on top of each stuffed pepper for added flavor.

7. Cover the baking dish with aluminum foil and bake in the preheated oven for 20-25 minutes, or until the peppers are tender.

8. Once cooked, remove the foil and let the stuffed peppers cool for a few minutes before serving.

9. Garnish with sliced olives and chopped parsley, if desired, and enjoy!

Zucchini Noodles with Pesto and Shrimp

Cooking Time: 10-15 minutes

Servings: 4

Ingredients

- 4 medium zucchinis
- 1 lb shrimp, peeled and deveined
- 1 cup fresh basil leaves
- ¼ cup pine nuts
- ¼ cup grated Parmesan cheese
- 2 cloves garlic, minced
- ¼ cup extra virgin olive oil
- Salt and pepper to taste
- Cherry tomatoes for garnish (optional)

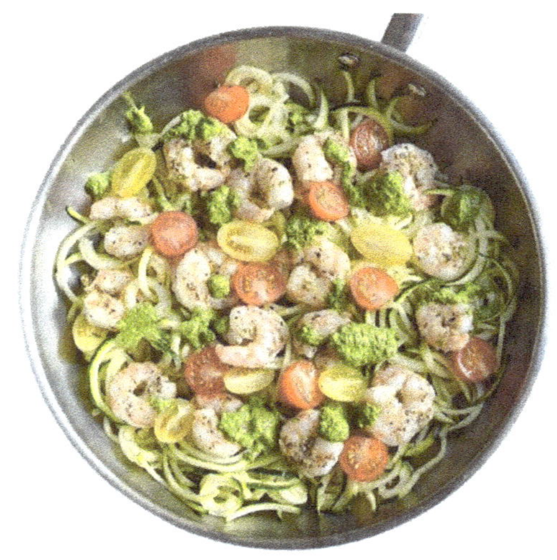

Procedure

1. Using a spiralizer or vegetable peeler, turn the zucchinis into noodles. Set aside.

2. In a food processor or blender, combine the basil leaves, pine nuts, Parmesan cheese, minced garlic, and olive oil. Blend until smooth to make the pesto sauce. Season with salt and pepper to taste.

3. Heat a skillet over medium heat. Add the shrimp and cook for 2-3 minutes on each side, until pink and cooked through. Remove the shrimp from the skillet and set aside.

4. In the same skillet, add the zucchini noodles and cook for 2-3 minutes, tossing occasionally, until just tender.

5. Add the cooked shrimp back to the skillet with the zucchini noodles. Pour the pesto sauce over the noodles and shrimp, stirring gently to coat everything evenly.

6. Cook for an additional 1-2 minutes, until everything is heated through.

7. Garnish with halved cherry tomatoes for added flavor and color (optional).

8. Serve hot and enjoy your delicious zucchini noodles with pesto and shrimp!

Egg Salad Lettuce Wraps

Cooking Time: 15 minutes (includes time for boiling eggs)

Servings: 4

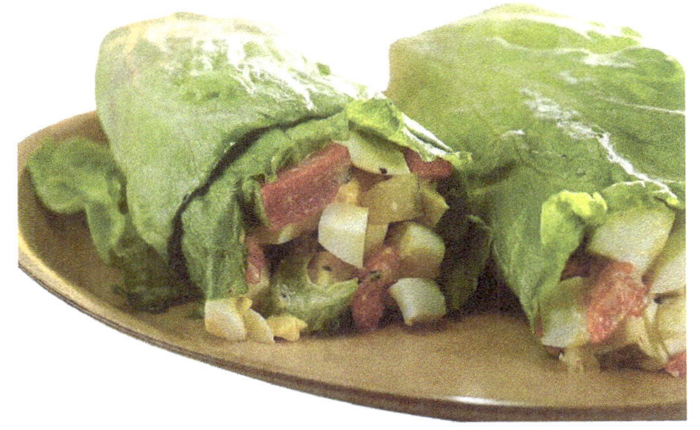

Ingredients

- 6 hard-boiled eggs, peeled and chopped
- ¼ cup mayonnaise
- 1 tablespoon Dijon mustard
- 2 tablespoons chopped chives or green onions
- Salt and pepper to taste
- 8 large lettuce leaves (such as butter lettuce or romaine)

Optional toppings: sliced avocado, diced tomatoes, cooked bacon pieces

Procedure

1. In a mixing bowl, combine the chopped hard-boiled eggs, mayonnaise, Dijon mustard, and chopped chives or green onions. Mix until well combined.
2. Season the egg salad with salt and pepper to taste, adjusting according to preference.
3. Lay out the lettuce leaves on a clean surface. Spoon the egg salad mixture onto each lettuce leaf, dividing it evenly among them.

4. Top each lettuce wrap with sliced avocado, diced tomatoes, or cooked bacon pieces for extra flavor and texture (optional).
5. Gently roll up each lettuce leaf, enclosing the egg salad filling.
6. Serve immediately and enjoy your delicious egg salad lettuce wraps!

Greek Salad with Grilled Lamb

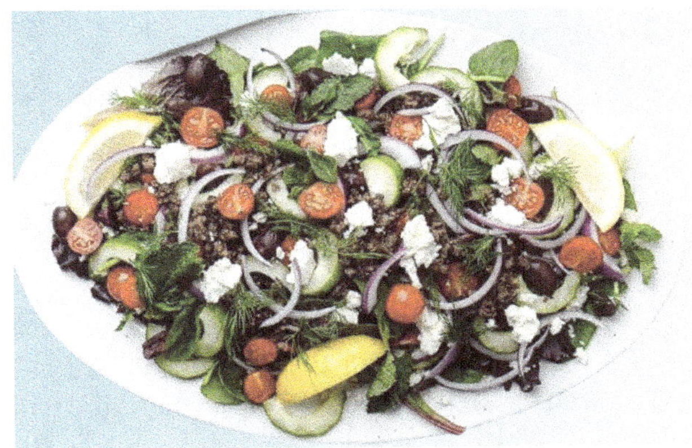

Cooking Time: 10-15 minutes

Servings: 4

Ingredients

- 1 lb lamb chops or lamb loin chops
- 1 tablespoon olive oil
- 1 teaspoon dried oregano
- Salt and pepper to taste
- 4 cups mixed salad greens (such as lettuce, spinach, or arugula)
- 1 cucumber, diced
- 1 cup cherry tomatoes, halved
- ½ red onion, thinly sliced
- ½ cup Kalamata olives
- ½ cup crumbled feta cheese
- Lemon wedges for garnish (optional)

For the dressing:

- ¼ cup extra virgin olive oil
- 2 tablespoons red wine vinegar
- 1 teaspoon dried oregano
- Salt and pepper to taste

Procedure

1. Preheat a grill or grill pan over medium-high heat.
2. In a small bowl, combine the olive oil, dried oregano, salt, and pepper. Rub the mixture all over the lamb chops.
3. Place the lamb chops on the preheated grill and cook for 3-4 minutes per side, or until desired doneness is reached.

Remove from the grill and let rest for a
few minutes before slicing.

4. Meanwhile, prepare the salad by
    combining the mixed greens, diced
    cucumber, halved cherry tomatoes,
    sliced red onion, Kalamata olives, and
    crumbled feta cheese in a large salad
    bowl.

5. In a small jar or bowl, whisk together
    the extra virgin olive oil, red wine
    vinegar, dried oregano, salt, and
    pepper to make the dressing.

6. Drizzle the dressing over the salad and
    toss gently to coat everything evenly.

7. Divide the salad among serving plates
    and top each with slices of grilled
    lamb.

8. Garnish with lemon wedges for a
   burst of freshness (optional).

9. Serve immediately and enjoy your
   Greek salad with grilled lamb!

Cobb Salad

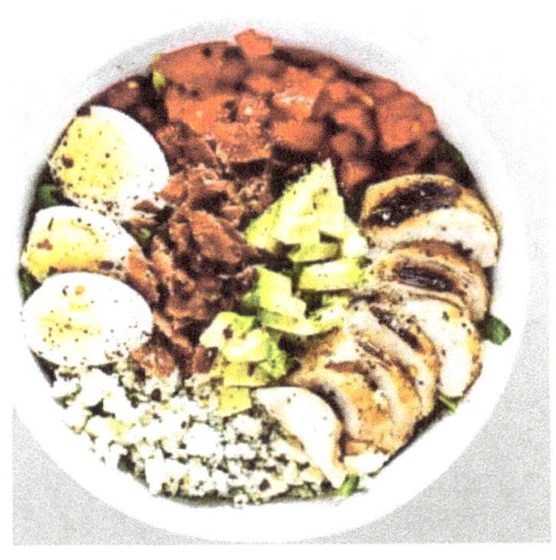

Cooking Time: 20 minutes (includes time for
boiling eggs and cooking bacon)

Servings: 4

<u>**Ingredients**</u>

- 4 cups mixed salad greens (such as lettuce, spinach, or arugula)
- 2 cooked chicken breasts, diced
- 4 hard-boiled eggs, chopped
- 4 slices cooked bacon, crumbled
- 1 avocado, diced
- 1 cup cherry tomatoes, halved
- ½ cup crumbled blue cheese or feta cheese
- Sliced green onions for garnish (optional)

For the dressing:

- ¼ cup olive oil

- 2 tablespoons red wine vinegar

- 1 teaspoon Dijon mustard

- Salt and pepper to taste

Procedure

1. In a large salad bowl, arrange the mixed salad greens as the base of the salad.

2. Arrange the diced chicken breast, chopped hard-boiled eggs, crumbled bacon, diced avocado, halved cherry tomatoes, and crumbled blue cheese on top of the mixed greens in rows or sections.

3. In a small jar or bowl, whisk together the olive oil, red wine vinegar, Dijon

mustard, salt, and pepper to make the dressing.

4. Drizzle the dressing over the Cobb salad.

5. Garnish with sliced green onions for added flavor and presentation (optional)

6. Serve immediately and enjoy your delicious Cobb salad!

Grilled Steak with Garlic Butter

Cooking Time: 10-12 minutes (adjust based on steak thickness and desired doneness).

Servings: 2

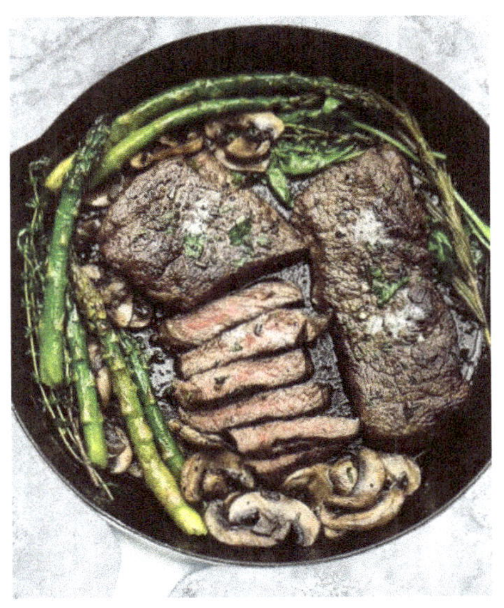

Ingredients

- 2 boneless ribeye steaks (about 8 oz each)
- Salt and pepper to taste
- 2 tbsp olive oil

Garlic Butter:

- 4 tbsp unsalted butter, softened
- 3 cloves garlic, minced
- 1 tbsp fresh parsley, chopped
- Salt to taste

Procedure

1. Preheat your grill to medium-high heat.
2. Season the steaks with salt, pepper, and a light drizzle of olive oil. Allow them to come to room temperature for 15 minutes.
3. While the steaks are resting, prepare the garlic butter. Mix together the softened butter, minced garlic, chopped parsley, and a pinch of salt. Set aside.

4. Place the steaks on the preheated grill and cook for about 4-5 minutes per side for medium-rare, adjusting the time based on your desired doneness.

5. During the last minute of grilling, spread a generous amount of the garlic butter over each steak. This adds a rich flavor and keeps the meat moist.

6. Remove the steaks from the grill and let them rest for a few minutes.

7. Top each steak with an extra dollop of garlic butter before serving.

Zoodle Carbonara

Cooking Time: 15 minutes.

Servings: 2

Ingredients

- 2 medium zucchinis
- 4 slices bacon, chopped
- 2 cloves garlic, minced
- 2 large eggs
- ½ cup grated Parmesan cheese
- Salt and pepper to taste
- Chopped parsley for garnish (optional)

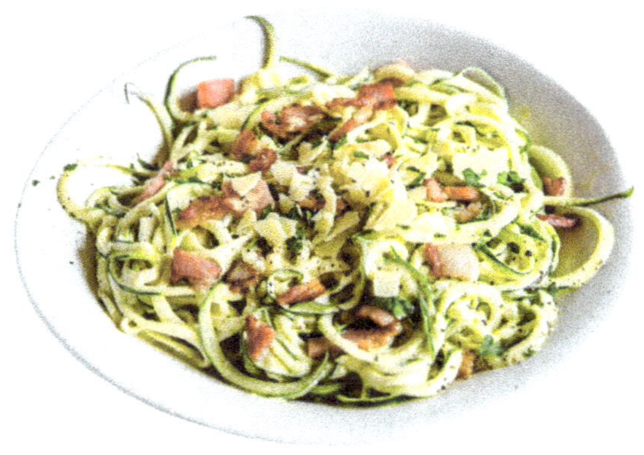

Procedure

1. Using a spiralizer, spiralize the zucchinis into zoodles (zucchini noodles). Set aside.

2. In a large skillet, cook the chopped bacon over medium heat until crispy. Remove the bacon from the skillet and set aside, leaving the bacon fat in the pan.

3. In the same skillet with the bacon fat, add the minced garlic and sauté for about 1 minute until fragrant.

4. Add the zucchini noodles to the skillet and toss to coat them in the bacon fat and garlic. Cook for about 2-3 minutes until the zoodles are just tender but still firm.

5. In a small bowl, whisk together the eggs and grated Parmesan cheese. Season with salt and pepper to taste.

6. Pour the egg and cheese mixture over the zucchini noodles in the skillet. Quickly toss everything together until the zoodles are coated evenly and the egg mixture thickens slightly.

7. Return the cooked bacon to the skillet and toss everything together once more.

8. Remove the skillet from the heat and garnish with chopped parsley if desired.

9. Divide the zoodle carbonara onto plates and serve immediately.

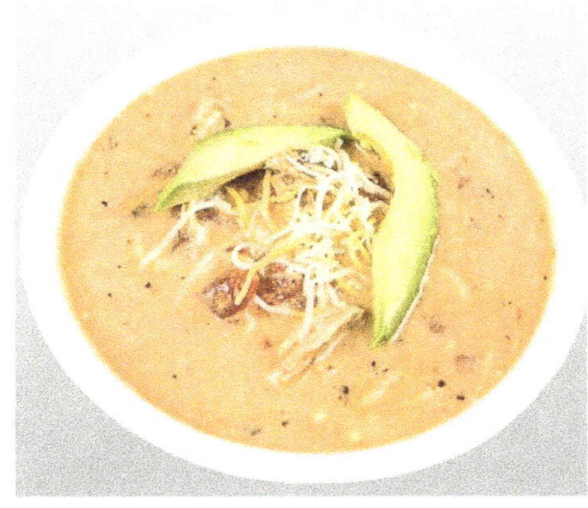

Mexican Chicken Soup

Cooking Time:

30 minutes.

Servings: 4

<u>Ingredients</u>

- 2 boneless, skinless chicken breasts
- 4 cups chicken broth
- 1 can (14.5 oz) diced tomatoes
- ½ cup diced onion
- ½ cup diced bell pepper (any color)
- ½ cup diced celery
- 2 cloves garlic, minced

- 1 tsp ground cumin
- ½ tsp chili powder
- Salt and pepper to taste

Optional toppings: sliced avocado, shredded cheese, chopped cilantro, lime wedges

Procedure

1. In a large pot, combine the chicken broth, diced tomatoes (with their juices), diced onion, diced bell pepper, diced celery, minced garlic, ground cumin, and chili powder. Stir to combine.

2. Add the boneless, skinless chicken breasts to the pot. Bring the soup to a boil over medium-high heat.

3. Once boiling, reduce the heat to low and cover the pot. Let the soup simmer for about 20-25 minutes, or until the chicken is cooked through and tender.

4. Once the chicken is cooked, remove it from the pot and shred it using two forks. Return the shredded chicken to the pot.

5. Season the soup with salt and pepper to taste, adjusting the seasoning as needed.

6. Serve the Mexican chicken soup hot, garnished with optional toppings such

as sliced avocado, shredded cheese, chopped cilantro, and lime wedges.

7. Ladle the soup into bowls and add desired toppings before serving.

Broccoli and Cheddar Stuffed Pork Chops

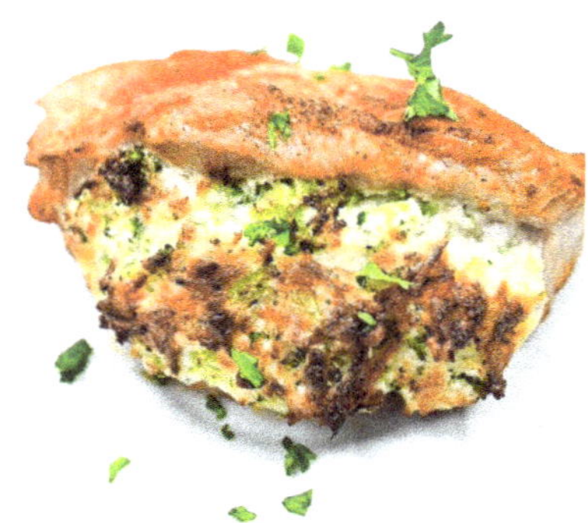

Cooking Time:
25-30 minutes.

Servings: 4

Ingredients

- 4 boneless pork chops (about 6 oz each)

- Salt and pepper to taste
- 1 cup cooked broccoli, chopped
- ½ cup shredded cheddar cheese
- 2 tbsp olive oil

Procedure

1. Preheat your oven to 375°F (190°C).
2. Using a sharp knife, carefully cut a pocket into each pork chop by slicing horizontally through the side, being careful not to cut all the way through.
3. Season the inside of each pork chop pocket with salt and pepper.
4. In a small bowl, mix together the chopped broccoli and shredded cheddar cheese.

5. Stuff each pork chop pocket with the broccoli and cheddar mixture, pressing gently to pack it in.

6. Heat olive oil in a large oven-safe skillet over medium-high heat.

7. Once the skillet is hot, add the stuffed pork chops and sear for about 3-4 minutes on each side until golden brown.

8. Transfer the skillet to the preheated oven and bake the pork chops for 15-20 minutes, or until the internal temperature reaches 145°F (63°C) for medium doneness.

9. Remove the skillet from the oven and let the pork chops rest for a few minutes.

10. Serve the broccoli and cheddar stuffed pork chops hot, with your choice of side dishes like steamed vegetables or a salad.

Spaghetti Squash with Meat Sauce

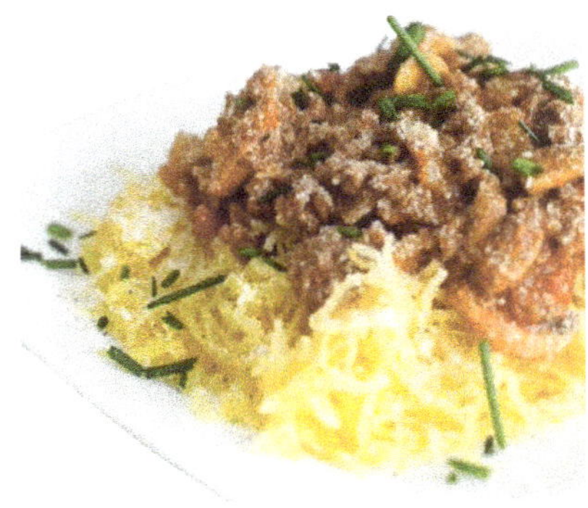

Cooking Time: 45-50 minutes.

Servings: 4

Ingredients

- 1 medium spaghetti squash

- 1 lb ground beef or turkey
- 1 can (14.5 oz) diced tomatoes
- ½ cup tomato sauce
- 2 cloves garlic, minced
- 1 tsp Italian seasoning
- Salt and pepper to taste
- Grated Parmesan cheese for garnish (optional)
- Chopped fresh basil for garnish (optional)

Procedure

1. Preheat your oven to 400°F (200°C).
2. Cut the spaghetti squash in half lengthwise and scoop out the seeds and pulp using a spoon.

3. Place the spaghetti squash halves, cut side down, on a baking sheet lined with parchment paper or aluminum foil.

4. Bake the spaghetti squash in the preheated oven for 35-45 minutes, or until the flesh is tender and easily pierced with a fork.

5. While the spaghetti squash is baking, prepare the meat sauce. In a large skillet, cook the ground beef or turkey over medium heat until browned and cooked through.

6. Add the minced garlic to the skillet with the cooked meat and cook for an additional 1-2 minutes until fragrant.

7. Stir in the diced tomatoes, tomato sauce, Italian seasoning, salt, and

pepper. Allow the sauce to simmer for 10-15 minutes, stirring occasionally, to allow the flavors to meld together.

8. Once the spaghetti squash is cooked, remove it from the oven and use a fork to scrape the flesh into spaghetti-like strands.

9. Serve the spaghetti squash topped with the meat sauce. Garnish with grated Parmesan cheese and chopped fresh basil if desired.

10. Serve the spaghetti squash with meat sauce hot, as a nutritious and satisfying low-carb meal option.

Turkey and Kale Soup

Cooking Time: 25-30 minutes.

Servings: 4

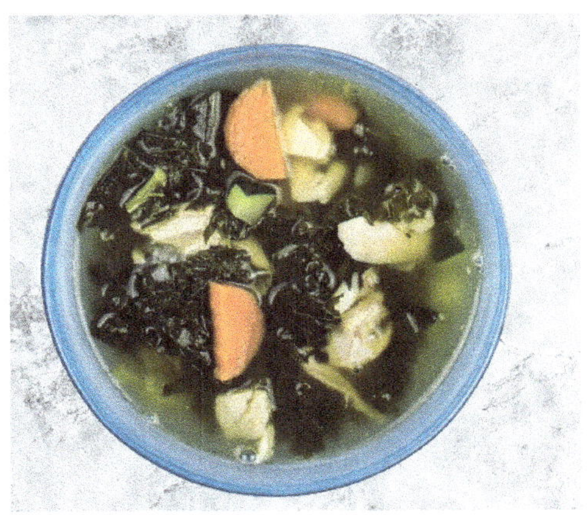

<u>Ingredients</u>

- 1 lb ground turkey
- 1 onion, chopped
- 2 cloves garlic, minced
- 4 cups chicken broth
- 1 can (14.5 oz) diced tomatoes
- 2 cups chopped kale leaves

- 1 tsp dried thyme
- Salt and pepper to taste
- Olive oil for cooking

Procedure

1. In a large pot, heat a drizzle of olive oil over medium heat. Add the chopped onion and minced garlic, and cook until softened and fragrant, about 3-4 minutes.
2. Add the ground turkey to the pot and cook, breaking it apart with a spoon, until browned and cooked through.

3. Pour in the chicken broth and diced tomatoes (with their juices). Stir to combine.

4. Add the chopped kale leaves and dried thyme to the pot. Stir well to incorporate.

5. Bring the soup to a simmer and let it cook for about 15-20 minutes, allowing the flavors to meld together and the kale to soften.

6. Season the soup with salt and pepper to taste, adjusting as needed.

7. Once the soup is cooked and seasoned to your liking, remove it from the heat.

8. Serve the turkey and kale soup hot, garnished with a sprinkle of freshly ground black pepper if desired.

9. Ladle the soup into bowls and serve immediately as a nutritious and comforting meal.

Zucchini and Parmesan Soup

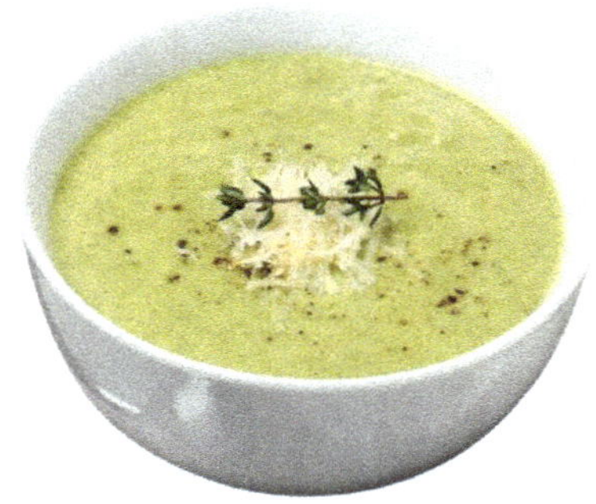

Cooking Time: 25-30 minutes.

Servings: 4

<u>Ingredients</u>

- 4 medium zucchinis, chopped

- 1 onion, chopped
- 2 cloves garlic, minced
- 4 cups chicken or vegetable broth
- ½ cup grated Parmesan cheese
- 2 tbsp olive oil
- Salt and pepper to taste
- Chopped fresh basil or parsley for garnish (optional)

Procedure

1. In a large pot, heat olive oil over medium heat. Add the chopped onion and minced garlic, and cook until softened and fragrant, about 3-4 minutes.
2. Add the chopped zucchinis to the pot and cook for another 5 minutes,

stirring occasionally, until they start to
soften.

3. Pour in the chicken or vegetable
    broth, enough to cover the zucchinis.
    Bring the mixture to a simmer.

4. Let the soup simmer for about 15-20
    minutes, or until the zucchinis are
    tender and cooked through.

5. Using an immersion blender or
    regular blender, puree the soup until
    smooth and creamy.

6. Stir in the grated Parmesan cheese
    until melted and incorporated into the
    soup.

7. Season the soup with salt and pepper
    to taste, adjusting as needed.

8. If desired, garnish the soup with
    chopped fresh basil or parsley.

9. Ladle the zucchini and Parmesan soup
    into bowls and serve hot, as a
    comforting and low-carb meal option.

Turkey Jerky

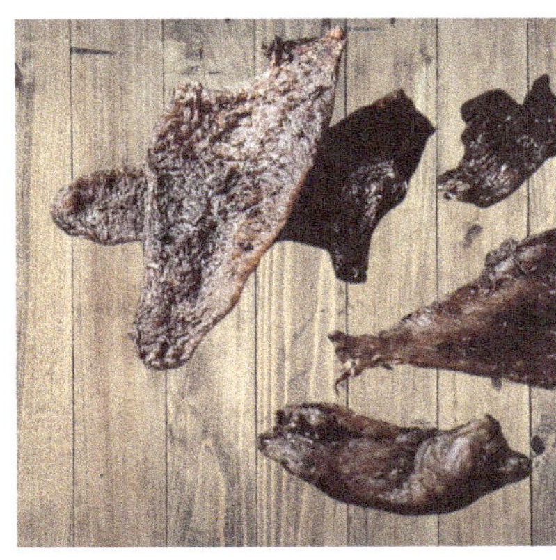

Cooking Time: 3-4

hours

Servings: 4

Ingredients

- 1 lb (450 g) turkey breast, thinly sliced

- ¼ cup (60 ml) soy sauce (low-sodium preferred)
- 2 tablespoons (30 ml) Worcestershire sauce
- 1 tablespoon (15 ml) apple cider vinegar
- 1 teaspoon (5 ml) liquid smoke
- 1 teaspoon (5 ml) garlic powder
- 1 teaspoon (5 ml) onion powder
- ½ teaspoon (2.5 ml) black pepper
- ½ teaspoon (2.5 ml) smoked paprika (optional)
- Cooking spray

Procedure

1. In a mixing bowl, combine soy sauce, Worcestershire sauce, apple cider

vinegar, liquid smoke, garlic powder, onion powder, black pepper, and smoked paprika (if using). Stir well to combine.

2. Add the thinly sliced turkey breast to the marinade, making sure each slice is evenly coated. Cover the bowl with plastic wrap and refrigerate for at least 2 hours or overnight for best results.

3. Preheat your oven to 175°F (80°C). Line a baking sheet with parchment paper and lightly coat it with cooking spray.

4. Remove the marinated turkey slices from the refrigerator and drain off any excess marinade. Place the slices in a

single layer on the prepared baking sheet.

5. Bake the turkey slices in the preheated oven for 3-4 hours, or until they are dried and chewy, but not brittle. Check on the jerky periodically and rotate the baking sheet if necessary for even drying.

6. Once the turkey jerky is done, remove it from the oven and let it cool completely before serving or storing.

7. Store the turkey jerky in an airtight container at room temperature for up to 2 weeks, or in the refrigerator for longer shelf life.

Greek yogurt with raspberries

Servings: 2

Ingredients

- 1 cup (240 g) plain Greek yogurt (full-fat or low-fat, depending on preference)
- ½ cup (75 g) fresh raspberries
- 1 tablespoon (15 ml) sugar-free sweetener (optional)
- ½ teaspoon (2.5 ml) vanilla extract (optional)

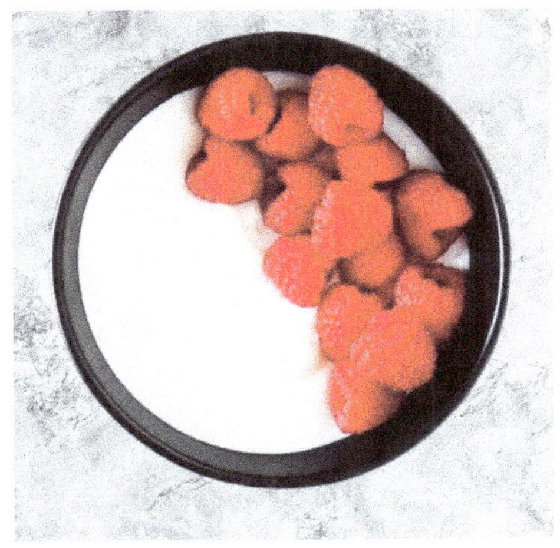

Procedure

1. In a bowl, combine the plain Greek yogurt with the sugar-free sweetener and vanilla extract (if using). Stir well to incorporate the sweetener and vanilla evenly into the yogurt.

2. Wash the fresh raspberries and gently pat them dry with a paper towel.

3. Spoon the sweetened Greek yogurt into serving bowls or glasses, dividing it evenly among the servings.

4. Top each portion of Greek yogurt with a generous serving of fresh raspberries.

5. Serve immediately and enjoy as a delicious and nutritious snack or dessert option.

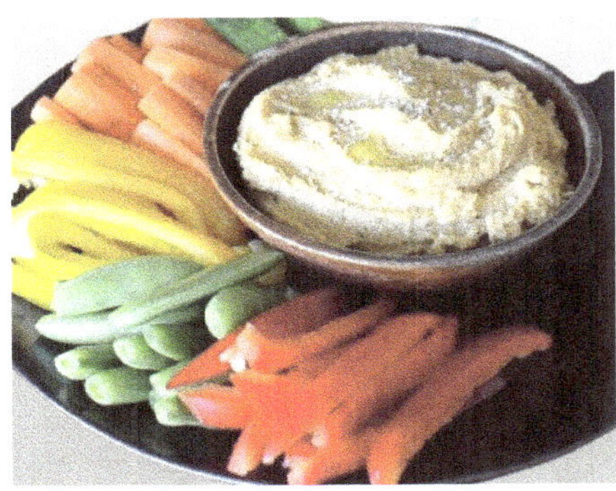

Servings: 4

Ingredients

- 2 bell peppers (choose a mix of colors for variety)
- 1 cup (240 g) hummus (store-bought or homemade)
- Fresh parsley, chopped, for garnish (optional)

Procedure

1. Wash and dry the bell peppers. Cut them into thin slices, removing seeds and membranes.
2. Arrange the sliced bell peppers on a serving platter or individual plates.
3. Place the hummus in a bowl and, if desired, garnish with chopped fresh parsley.
4. Serve the sliced bell peppers alongside the bowl of hummus, allowing individuals to dip the peppers into the hummus.

Deviled Eggs

Cooking Time: 10-12 minutes

Servings: 6

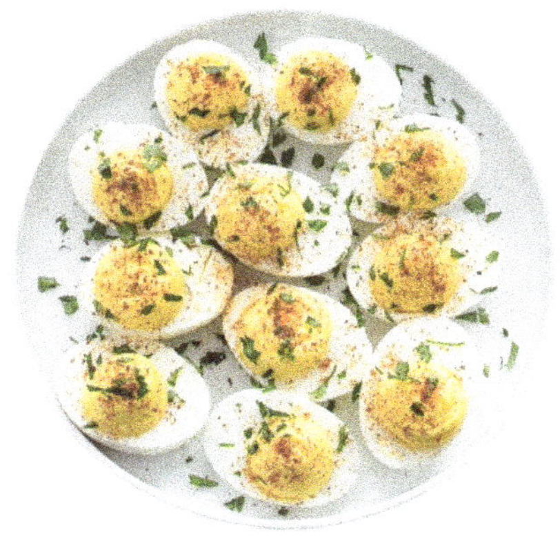

Ingredients

- 6 large eggs
- 2 tablespoons (30 g) mayonnaise (full-fat or low-fat, depending on preference)
- 1 teaspoon (5 ml) Dijon mustard
- ½ teaspoon (2.5 ml) white vinegar
- ¼ teaspoon (1.25 ml) salt
- ¼ teaspoon (1.25 ml) black pepper
- Paprika, for garnish

- Fresh chives or parsley, chopped, for garnish (optional)

Procedure

1. Place the eggs in a single layer in a saucepan and cover them with water, ensuring the water level is about an inch above the eggs.
2. Bring the water to a boil over medium-high heat. Once boiling, remove the saucepan from the heat, cover it with a lid, and let the eggs sit in the hot water for 10-12 minutes.
3. While the eggs are cooking, prepare a bowl of ice water. Once the eggs are done, immediately transfer them to

the ice water bath to cool for a few minutes.

4. Once the eggs are cool, carefully peel off the shells and slice each egg in half lengthwise. Gently remove the yolks and place them in a separate bowl.

5. Mash the egg yolks with a fork until they are finely crumbled.

6. To the mashed yolks, add mayonnaise, Dijon mustard, white vinegar, salt, and black pepper. Stir well to combine, ensuring a smooth and creamy consistency.

7. Spoon or pipe the yolk mixture back into the hollowed-out egg whites, dividing it evenly among the halves.

8. Sprinkle the deviled eggs with paprika for added flavor and garnish with

chopped fresh chives or parsley, if
desired.

9. Serve the deviled eggs immediately, or
refrigerate them for later enjoyment.

Cherry tomatoes with mozzarella

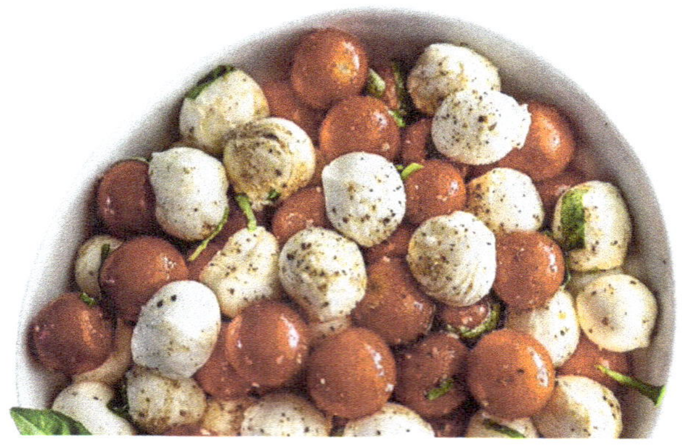

Servings: 4

Ingredients

- 1 pint (about 2 cups or 300 g) cherry tomatoes
- 8 oz (225 g) fresh mozzarella cheese, cut into bite-sized pieces
- Fresh basil leaves, torn or chopped
- Balsamic glaze, for drizzling (optional)
- Extra virgin olive oil, for drizzling
- Salt and black pepper, to taste

Procedure

1. Wash the cherry tomatoes and pat them dry with a paper towel. If desired, cut them in half for easier eating.
2. Place the cherry tomatoes and mozzarella cheese pieces in a serving bowl or on a platter.

3. Scatter torn or chopped fresh basil leaves over the cherry tomatoes and mozzarella.

4. Drizzle the cherry tomatoes and mozzarella with balsamic glaze (if using) and extra virgin olive oil.

5. Season with salt and black pepper to taste.

6. Gently toss the ingredients together to ensure they are evenly coated with the dressing and seasoning.

7. Serve immediately as a refreshing and flavorful appetizer or snack.

Peanut butter fat bombs

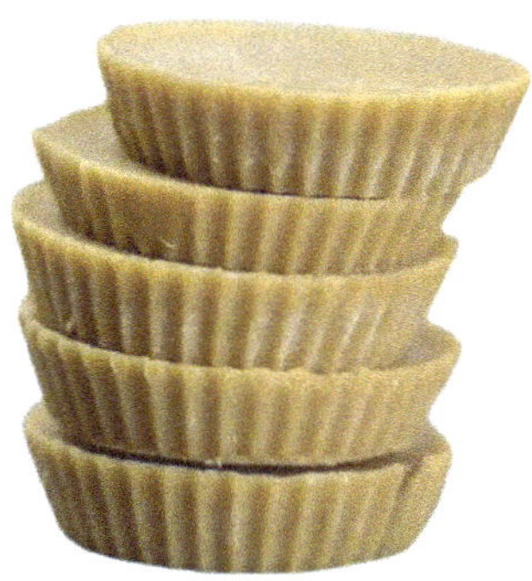

Cooking Time: 30 minutes (for setting in the freezer)

Servings: 12 fat bombs

Ingredients

- ½ cup (120 g) natural peanut butter (sugar-free)
- ¼ cup (56 g) coconut oil, melted
- 2 tablespoons (30 ml) heavy cream
- 1 tablespoon (15 ml) sugar-free sweetener (such as erythritol or stevia)
- ½ teaspoon (2.5 ml) vanilla extract
- Pinch of salt

<u>Procedure</u>

1. In a mixing bowl, combine the melted coconut oil, natural peanut butter, heavy cream, sugar-free sweetener, vanilla extract, and a pinch of salt. Stir well until smooth and thoroughly combined.

2. Line a mini muffin tin with mini
   muffin liners.

3. Pour the peanut butter mixture evenly
   into the mini muffin liners, filling
   each about halfway full.

4. Place the muffin tin in the freezer and
   let the fat bombs set for about 30
   minutes, or until firm.

5. Once firm, remove the fat bombs from
   the muffin tin and transfer them to an
   airtight container.

6. Store the peanut butter fat bombs in
   the refrigerator or freezer until ready
   to enjoy.

Keto Lemon Bars

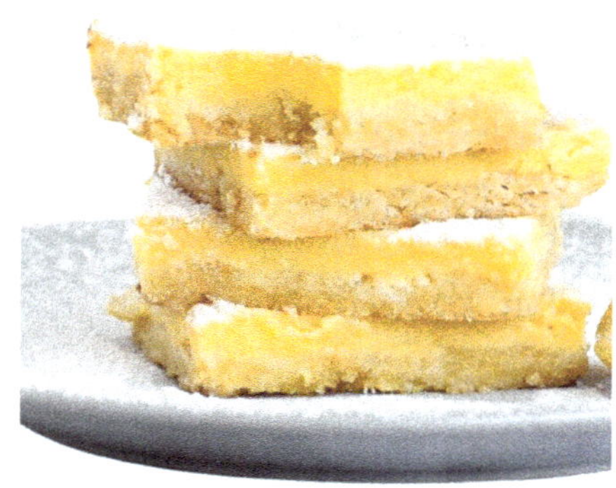

Cooking Time:

- 10-12 minutes (for crust)
- 20-25 minutes (for lemon filling)
- 2 hours (chilling time)

Servings: 16 small bars

Ingredients

For the Crust:

- 1 cup (100 g) almond flour
- ¼ cup (60 g) unsalted butter, melted
- 2 tablespoons (30 g) sugar-free sweetener (such as erythritol or stevia)
- Pinch of salt

For the Lemon Filling:

- 4 large eggs
- ½ cup (120 ml) fresh lemon juice
- 1 tablespoon (15 g) lemon zest
- 1 cup (200 g) sugar-free sweetener
- 2 tablespoons (15 g) coconut flour
- ½ teaspoon baking powder

- Powdered sugar-free sweetener for dusting (optional)

<u>**Procedure**</u>

For the Crust:

1. Preheat your oven to 350°F (175°C). Line an 8x8-inch (20x20 cm) baking dish with parchment paper, leaving some overhang for easy removal.
2. In a bowl, combine almond flour, melted butter, sugar-free sweetener, and a pinch of salt. Mix until well combined.
3. Press the mixture evenly into the bottom of the prepared baking dish to form the crust.

4. Bake the crust in the preheated oven
   for 10-12 minutes or until golden
   brown. Remove from the oven and let
   it cool slightly.

For the Lemon Filling:

5. In a separate bowl, whisk together
   eggs, fresh lemon juice, lemon zest,
   sugar-free sweetener, coconut flour,
   and baking powder until smooth.
6. Pour the lemon mixture over the
   baked crust.
7. Bake for an additional 20-25 minutes
   or until the filling is set.
8. Allow the lemon bars to cool in the
   baking dish, then refrigerate for at
   least 2 hours or until fully chilled.

9. Once chilled, use the parchment paper overhang to lift the lemon bars out of the dish. Cut into squares.
10. Optionally, dust with powdered sugar-free sweetener before serving.

Berry and whipped Cream Parfait

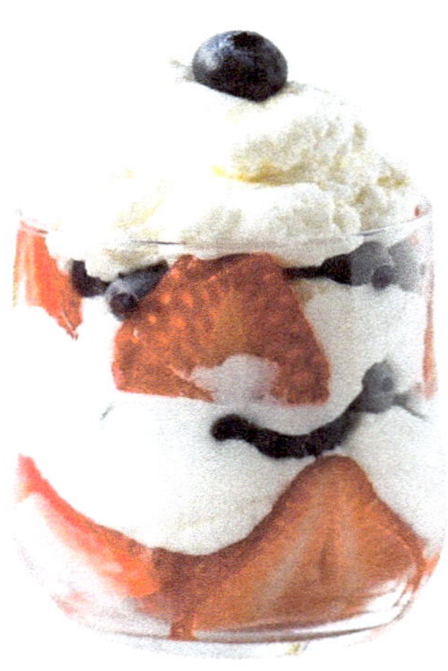

Servings: 2

Ingredients

- 1 cup (240 ml) heavy whipping cream

- 2 tablespoons (30 ml) sugar-free
  sweetener (such as erythritol or stevia)

- 1 teaspoon (5 ml) vanilla extract

- 1 cup (150 g) mixed berries (such as
  strawberries, blueberries, and
  raspberries)

- 1/4 cup (25 g) chopped nuts (optional,
  such as almonds or walnuts)

Procedure

1. In a mixing bowl, whip the heavy
   whipping cream using a hand mixer or
   stand mixer until stiff peaks form.

2. Add sugar-free sweetener and vanilla
   extract to the whipped cream and
   continue to beat until well combined.

3. Wash and dry the mixed berries. If using strawberries, remove the stems and slice them.

4. To assemble the parfaits, layer whipped cream, mixed berries, and chopped nuts (if using) in serving glasses or bowls.

5. Repeat the layers until the glasses are filled, ending with a dollop of whipped cream on top.

6. Garnish with a few whole berries or a sprinkle of chopped nuts for decoration.

7. Serve immediately and enjoy as a delicious and satisfying dessert or snack option.

Keto Cheesecake with Almond Crust

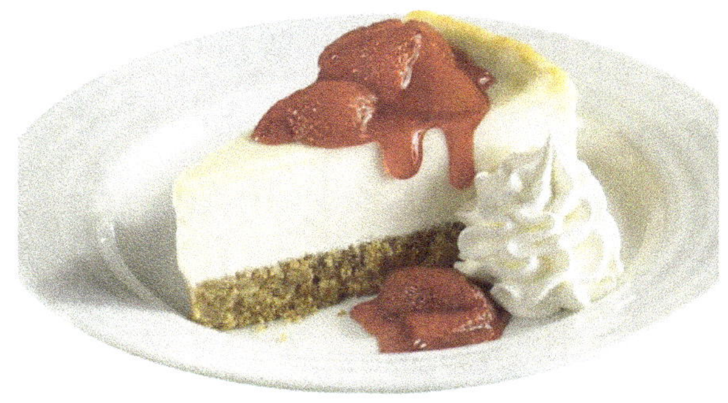

Cooking Time:

- 10-12 minutes (for crust)
- 45-50 minutes (for filling)
- 4 hours (chilling time)

Servings: 12

Ingredients

For the Almond Crust:

- 1½ cups (150 g) almond flour
- ¼ cup (50 g) unsalted butter, melted
- 2 tablespoons (30 g) sugar-free sweetener (such as erythritol or stevia)
- ½ teaspoon (2.5 ml) vanilla extract

For the Cheesecake Filling:

- 16 oz (450 g) cream cheese, softened
- ⅔ cup (160 ml) sour cream
- ⅔ cup (130 g) sugar-free sweetener
- 2 large eggs
- 1 teaspoon (5 ml) vanilla extract
- 1 tablespoon (15 ml) fresh lemon juice
- Pinch of salt

Procedure

For the Almond Crust:

1. Preheat your oven to 325°F (160°C). Grease a 9-inch (23 cm) springform pan with butter or cooking spray.
2. In a mixing bowl, combine almond flour, melted butter, sugar-free sweetener, and vanilla extract. Mix until well combined and a dough forms.
3. Press the dough evenly into the bottom of the prepared springform pan to form the crust.
4. Bake the crust in the preheated oven for 10-12 minutes, or until lightly golden brown. Remove from the oven and let it cool while preparing the filling.

For the Cheesecake Filling:

5. In a large mixing bowl, beat the softened cream cheese until smooth and creamy.
6. Add sour cream, sugar-free sweetener, eggs, vanilla extract, fresh lemon juice, and a pinch of salt to the cream cheese. Beat until well combined and smooth.
7. Pour the cheesecake filling over the cooled almond crust in the springform pan.
8. Smooth the top with a spatula to ensure an even layer.
9. Bake the cheesecake in the preheated oven for 45-50 minutes, or until the

edges are set and the center is slightly jiggly.

10. Turn off the oven and leave the cheesecake inside with the door closed for an additional 10 minutes.

11. Remove the cheesecake from the oven and let it cool to room temperature.

12. Once cooled, refrigerate the cheesecake for at least 4 hours or overnight to set.

13. Before serving, carefully run a knife around the edges of the cheesecake to loosen it from the pan.

14. Slice and serve the keto cheesecake with almond crust chilled, optionally garnished with fresh berries or whipped cream.

Sugar-free Jello with whipped Cream

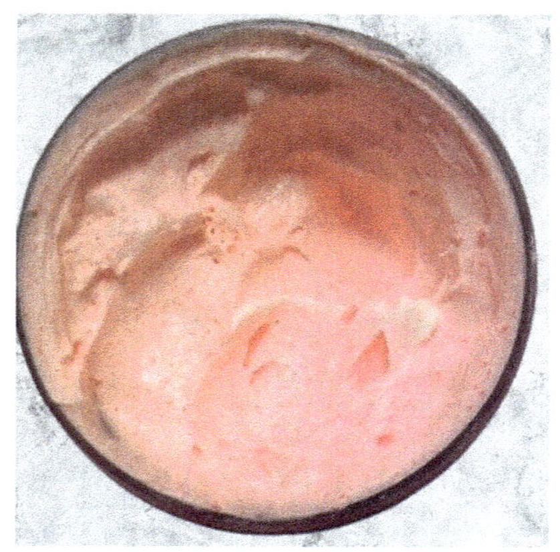

Cooking Time: 4 hours (chilling time for gelatin)

Servings: 4

Ingredients

- 1 (0.3 oz) package sugar-free flavored gelatin (such as Jello)
- 1 cup (240 ml) boiling water
- 1 cup (240 ml) cold water
- ½ cup (120 ml) heavy whipping cream
- 1 tablespoon (15 ml) sugar-free sweetener (such as erythritol or stevia)
- ½ teaspoon (2.5 ml) vanilla extract (optional)

Procedure

1. In a mixing bowl, dissolve the sugar-free flavored gelatin in boiling water, stirring until completely dissolved.
2. Stir in cold water until well combined.

3. Pour the gelatin mixture into serving cups or molds, filling each about halfway full.

4. Refrigerate the gelatin cups for at least 4 hours, or until firm and set.

5. In a separate mixing bowl, whip the heavy whipping cream until stiff peaks form.

6. Add sugar-free sweetener and vanilla extract (if using) to the whipped cream, and continue to beat until well combined.

7. Once the gelatin is set, top each cup with a dollop of whipped cream.

8. Serve immediately and enjoy as a refreshing and guilt-free dessert option.

DRINKS RECIPES

Iced herbal tea with lemon

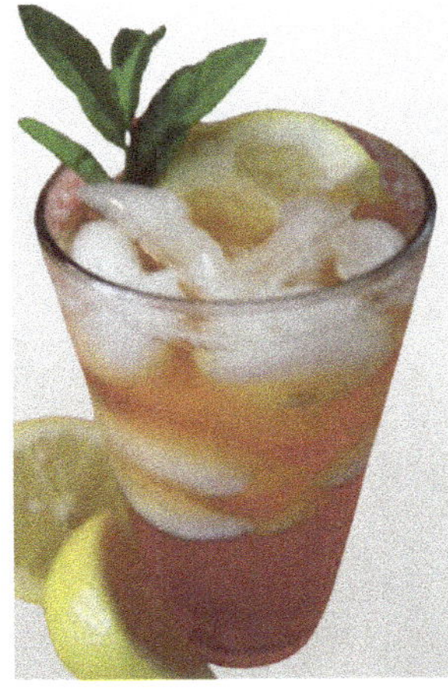

Cooking Time: 5-7

minutes (steeping time)

Servings: 4

<u>Ingredients</u>

- 4 cups (960 ml) water
- 4 herbal tea bags (such as chamomile, peppermint, or herbal blend)
- 1 lemon, sliced

- Sugar-free sweetener (optional)
- Ice cubes

Procedure

1. Bring 4 cups of water to a boil in a saucepan or kettle.
2. Once boiling, remove the water from heat and add the herbal tea bags to the hot water.
3. Let the tea bags steep in the hot water for about 5-7 minutes, depending on the desired strength of the tea.
4. After steeping, remove the tea bags from the water and discard them.
5. Allow the brewed tea to cool to room temperature, then transfer it to a pitcher.

6. Add slices of lemon to the pitcher of tea, stirring to combine.

7. Taste the tea and add sugar-free sweetener if desired, adjusting to your preferred level of sweetness.

8. Refrigerate the iced herbal tea until chilled, or add ice cubes to serve immediately over ice.

9. Serve the iced herbal tea with lemon in glasses, garnishing with additional lemon slices if desired.

Cucumber and mint infused water

Servings: 4

<u>Ingredients</u>

- 1 medium cucumber, washed and thinly sliced
- 8-10 fresh mint leaves, washed
- 4 cups (960 ml) water
- Ice cubes

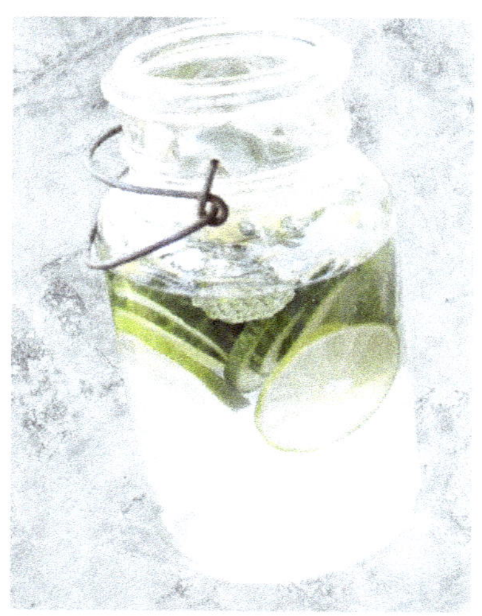

Procedure

1. In a pitcher, add the thinly sliced cucumber and fresh mint leaves.

2. Pour 4 cups of water into the pitcher, covering the cucumber slices and mint leaves.

3. Stir gently to distribute the cucumber and mint throughout the water.

4. Cover the pitcher and refrigerate for at least 2 hours, or preferably overnight, to allow the flavors to infuse.

5. When ready to serve, fill glasses with ice cubes.

6. Pour the cucumber and mint infused water into the glasses, ensuring each glass has some cucumber slices and mint leaves.

7. Serve the refreshing infused water immediately and enjoy!

Bone broth

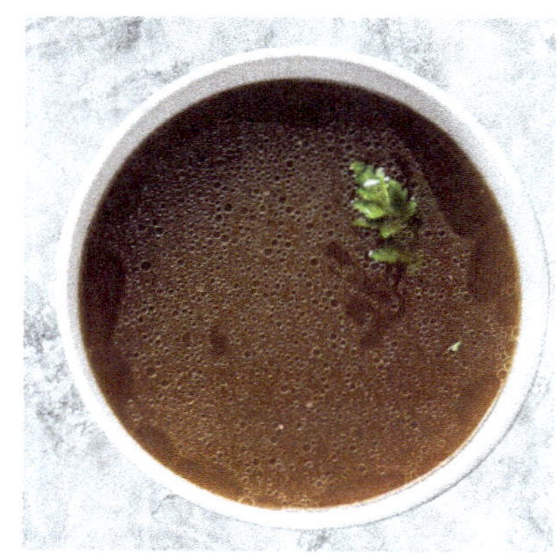

Cooking Time: 4-24
hours

Servings: 10

<u>Ingredients</u>

- 2-3 lbs (900-1350 g) beef bones, chicken carcass, or a combination of bones
- 2 carrots, washed and roughly chopped
- 2 celery stalks, washed and roughly chopped
- 1 onion, peeled and quartered

- 4 cloves garlic, smashed

- 2 bay leaves

- 1 tablespoon (15 ml) apple cider vinegar

- Salt and pepper, to taste

- Water, enough to cover the bones and vegetables

Procedure

1. Preheat your oven to 400°F (200°C).

2. Place the bones on a baking sheet and roast them in the preheated oven for 30-40 minutes, or until they are browned and fragrant.

3. Transfer the roasted bones to a large stockpot or slow cooker.

4. Add chopped carrots, celery, onion, smashed garlic cloves, bay leaves, apple cider vinegar, salt, and pepper to the pot or slow cooker.

5. Fill the pot or slow cooker with enough water to cover the bones and vegetables.

6. If using a stockpot, bring the mixture to a boil over high heat. Once boiling, reduce the heat to low and let the broth simmer, partially covered, for at least 4 hours, up to 24 hours. If using a slow cooker, set it to low heat and let the broth cook for 8-24 hours.

7. As the broth simmers, skim off any foam or impurities that rise to the surface with a spoon.

8. Once the broth has simmered for the desired time, remove the bones and vegetables from the pot or slow cooker using a slotted spoon or strainer.

9. Strain the broth through a fine-mesh sieve or cheesecloth into a clean container to remove any remaining solids.

10. Let the broth cool to room temperature, then refrigerate it for up to 5 days, or freeze it for longer storage.

Keto-friendly protein shakes

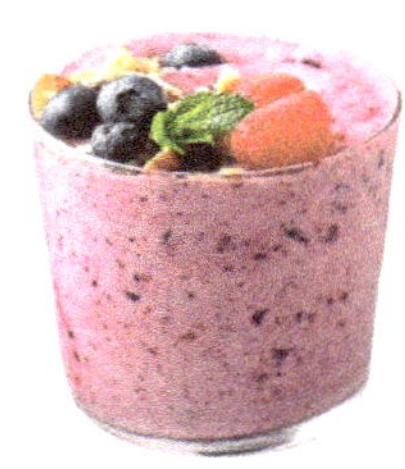

Servings: 1

<u>**Ingredients**</u>

- 1 cup (240 ml) unsweetened almond milk or coconut milk
- 1 scoop (about 25-30 g) of your favorite low-carb protein powder (such as whey protein isolate or plant-based protein)
- 1 tablespoon (15 g) almond butter or peanut butter (sugar-free and natural)
- ½ cup (75 g) frozen berries (such as strawberries, blueberries, or raspberries)
- ¼ teaspoon (1.25 ml) vanilla extract
- Optional: sugar-free sweetener to taste (such as erythritol or stevia)
- Ice cubes

<u>**Procedure**</u>

1. In a blender, combine unsweetened almond milk or coconut milk, low-carb protein powder, almond butter or peanut butter, frozen berries, vanilla extract, and optional sugar-free sweetener to taste.

2. Add a handful of ice cubes to the blender to make the shake cold and refreshing.

3. Blend all the ingredients together until smooth and creamy, scraping down the sides of the blender if needed.

4. Taste the protein shake and adjust the sweetness or thickness by adding more sweetener or almond milk, if desired.

5. Once blended to your desired consistency, pour the keto-friendly protein shake into a glass and serve immediately.

CHAPTER FIVE

Tips and Tricks for Success on the Atkins Diet

There are a few tips and tricks that can help make the Atkins diet more successful. First, it's important to plan ahead and make sure you have healthy, low-carb options available when you're hungry. This will help you avoid temptation and make it easier to stick to the diet. One popular option is to make a trail mix of nuts, seeds, and unsweetened coconut flakes. You can also try celery sticks with peanut butter, or roasted chickpeas with salt and pepper. For a sweet treat, try berries with heavy cream or unsweetened Greek yogurt. There are endless possibilities for delicious and nutritious low-carb snacks. Just be sure to avoid processed, packaged snacks that are high in carbs and unhealthy fats.

Make sure you're eating plenty of protein and healthy fats to keep you satisfied and prevent cravings. You can make a keto-friendly chocolate mousse by blending avocado, cocoa powder, and a little bit of stevia or monk fruit sweetener. Or, you can make a "fat bomb" by combining coconut oil, nut butter, and a sweetener. These are great options for when you're craving something sweet but don't want to derail your diet.

One way to make meal planning easier is to batch cook your meals. For example, you could make a big batch of roasted veggies on the weekend, and then use them throughout the week in different meals. You could also cook a large batch of chicken or ground beef and use it in different recipes throughout the week. Meal planning will not only save you time, but it will also help you stay on track with your low-carb diet.

Finally, staying hydrated is important for overall health, but it's especially important when you're on a low-carb diet. That's because carbs retain water, so when you cut back on carbs, you'll naturally lose some water weight. This can lead to dehydration, so it's important to drink plenty of water.

Aim for at least eight glasses of water per day. You can also drink unsweetened herbal tea, coffee, or bone broth to get in your hydration. And remember to drink more water when it's hot outside or if you're exercising. Being well-hydrated will help you feel your best and stay on track with your low-carb diet.

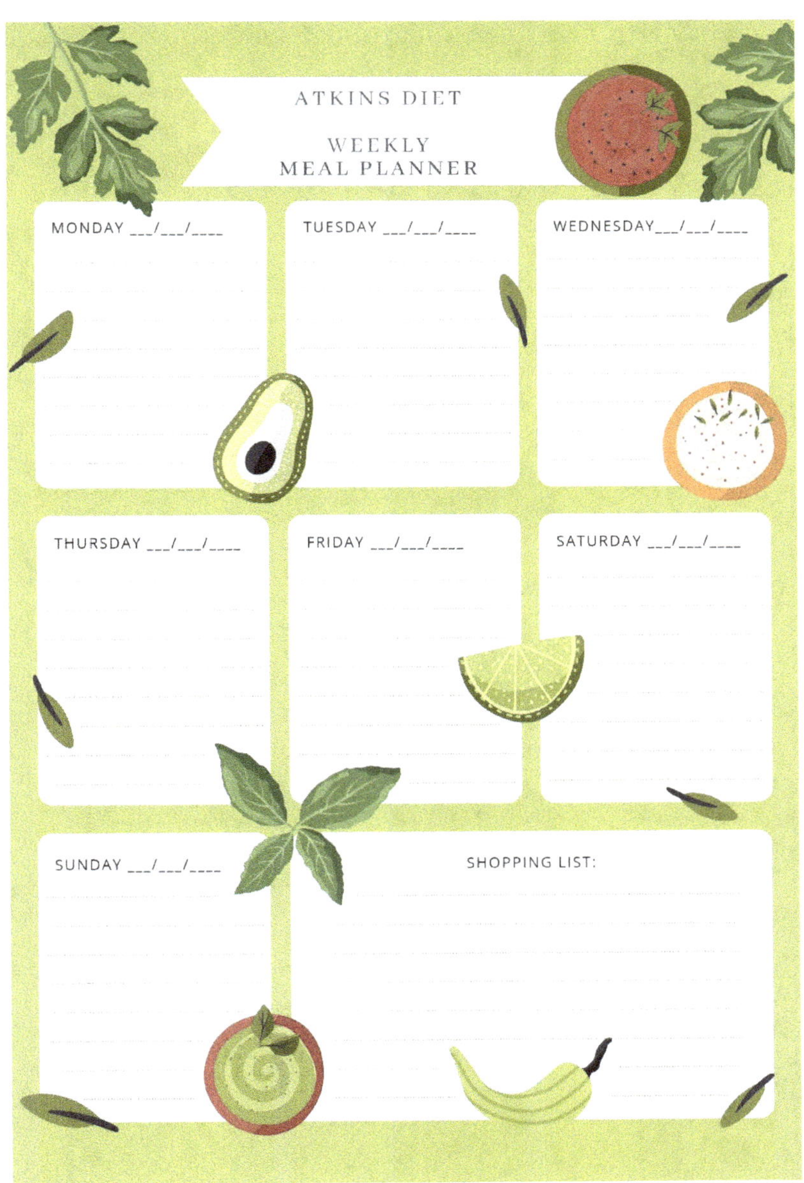

ATKINS DIET

WEEKLY
MEAL PLANNER

MONDAY ___/___/____

TUESDAY ___/___/____

WEDNESDAY___/___/____

THURSDAY ___/___/____

FRIDAY ___/___/____

SATURDAY ___/___/____

SUNDAY ___/___/____

SHOPPING LIST:

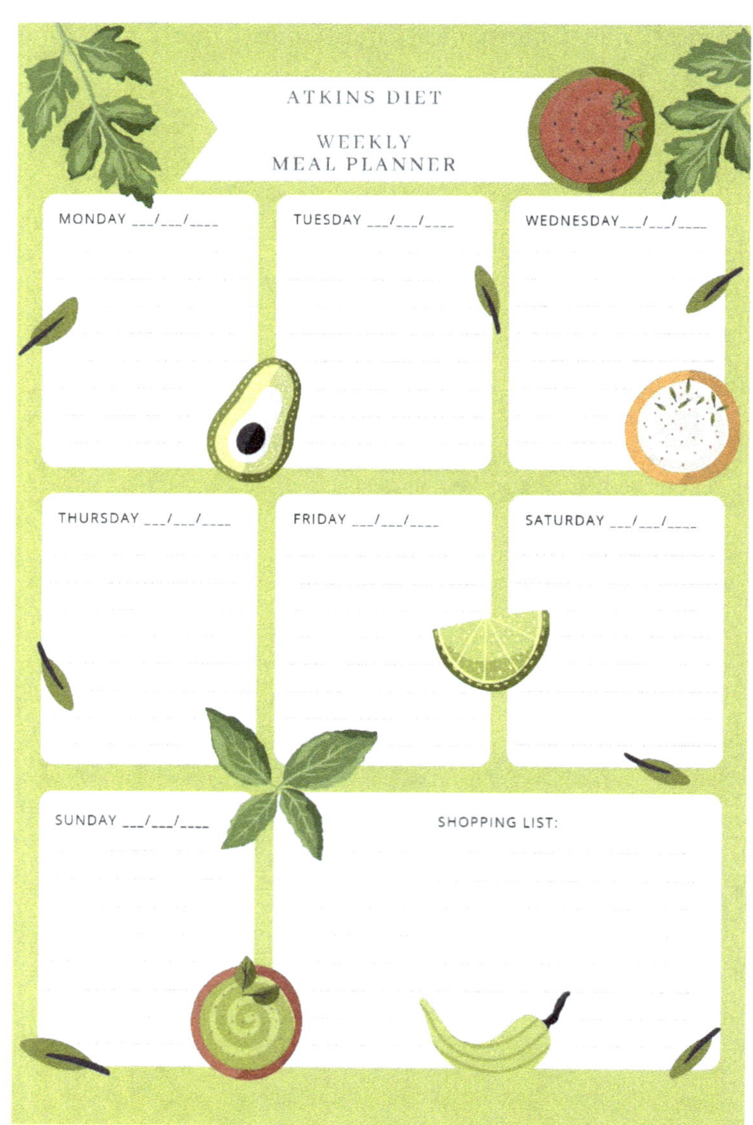

ATKINS DIET
WEEKLY
MEAL PLANNER

MONDAY ___/___/____

TUESDAY ___/___/____

WEDNESDAY___/___/____

THURSDAY ___/___/____

FRIDAY ___/___/____

SATURDAY ___/___/____

SUNDAY ___/___/____

SHOPPING LIST:

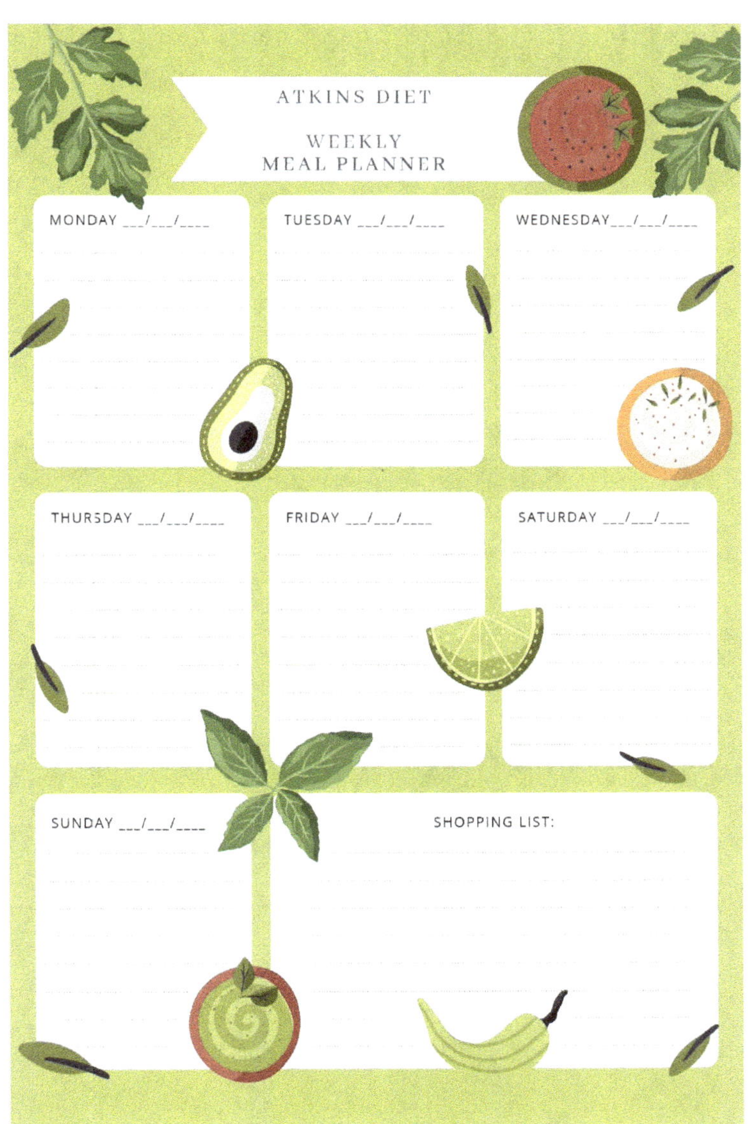

ATKINS DIET

WEEKLY
MEAL PLANNER

MONDAY ___/___/____

TUESDAY ___/___/____

WEDNESDAY___/___/____

THURSDAY ___/___/____

FRIDAY ___/___/____

SATURDAY ___/___/____

SUNDAY ___/___/____

SHOPPING LIST:

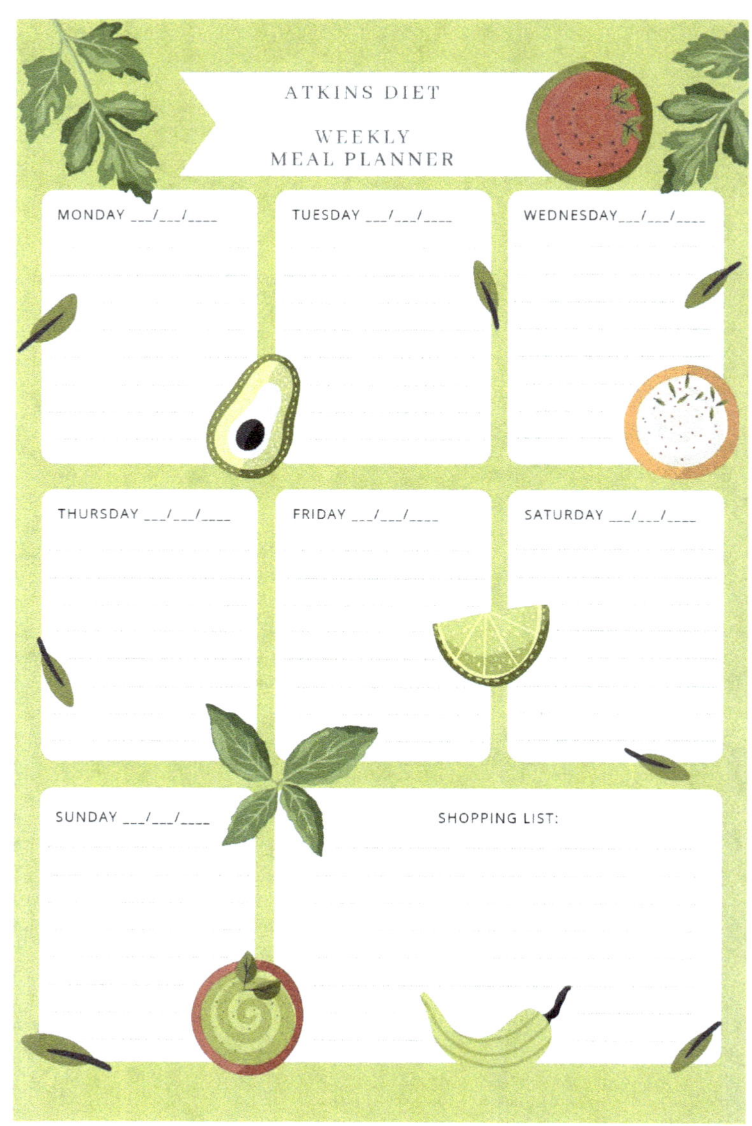

ATKINS DIET
WEEKLY
MEAL PLANNER
MONDAY ___/___/____
TUESDAY ___/___/____
WEDNESDAY___/___/____
THURSDAY ___/___/____
FRIDAY ___/___/____
SATURDAY ___/___/____
SUNDAY ___/___/____
SHOPPING LIST:

CONCLUSION

The Atkins diet is a great option for seniors who are looking to lose weight and improve their health. The diet is simple to follow and can be tailored to individual needs. With a little bit of planning and preparation, seniors can easily enjoy all the benefits that the Atkins diet has to offer. The diet can help seniors feel more energetic, lose weight, and reduce the risk of chronic diseases. So, if you're a senior looking to make a positive change in your life, consider giving the Atkins diet a try. You may be surprised at how easy it is to follow and how good you feel!

Remember, the key to success on any diet is finding what works for you and sticking with it. There's no one-size-fits-all solution, so don't be afraid to experiment and find what works best for you. Just be sure to listen to your body and consult with your doctor or dietitian before making any major changes to your diet. With the right approach, you can make the Atkins diet work for you and reach your health goals.